Healing Through Nutrition

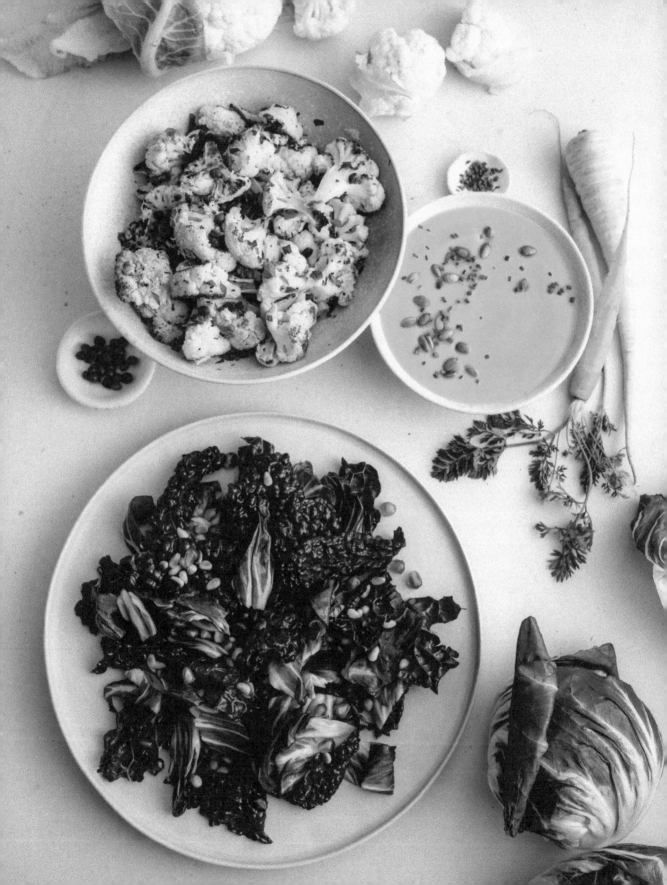

Healing
THROUGH
NUTRITION

THE ESSENTIAL GUIDE TO
50 PLANT-BASED
NUTRITIONAL SOURCES

ELIZA SAVAGE RD, MS, CDN

PHOTOGRAPHY BY *Annie Martin*

ROCKRIDGE
PRESS

Interior and Cover Designer: Linda Snorina
Art Producer: Sue Bischofberger
Editor: Crystal Nero
Production Manager: Riley Hoffman
Production Editor: Melissa Edeburn

Photography © 2019 Annie Martin. Food styling by Oscar Molinar.

Illustrations © Vecteezy.com. Food pyramid © BaeBae/iStock, p. 13.
Plate diagram © peanutpie/iStock, p. 13.

Author photo courtesy of Eric Striffler.

ISBN: Print 978-1-64152-813-9 | eBook 978-1-64152-814-6

R0

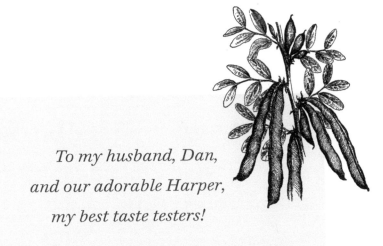

To my husband, Dan,
and our adorable Harper,
my best taste testers!

To all those looking to heal: May you find
health, happiness, and joy through food
and in all areas of your life.

CONTENTS

5 WHOLE GRAINS, LEGUMES, AND NUTS 101

6 HERBS AND SPICES 137

7 COFFEE AND TEA 171

INTRODUCTION

Let food be thy medicine!

Ever since I can remember, I've been interested in the healing powers of food. I spent many of my childhood years taking antibiotics and sitting out gym class and playground activities because of my life-threatening asthma and allergies. I lived in fear of the next asthma attack but yearned to be an athlete like my sister. As an alternative, my mom and dad encouraged me to share their love of cooking and to take an active role in the kitchen. I jumped in wholeheartedly. Soon I was roasting carrots, sautéing string beans, and baking chocolate chip cookies (with some oats thrown in for good measure). From these early culinary experiences, I developed a deep love for the art of cooking and cultivated an interest in food's influence of on how you feel.

As my recipe repertoire expanded, my asthma eventually improved, and my desire to become an athlete became a reality. I joined my high school's cross-country team and, let's just say, I've been running ever since! Although healthy eating was always a priority, bagels and Gatorade fueled most of my runs throughout high school and college. When I moved to New York City after graduation and started training for my first marathon, I quickly realized I needed to change my nutrition strategy. Cue the salads, smoothies, and soups! I said sayonara to artificial sweeteners, cut down on simple carbohydrates, and started cooking more frequently in my tiny apartment. If it came from the ground, it was in my kitchen!

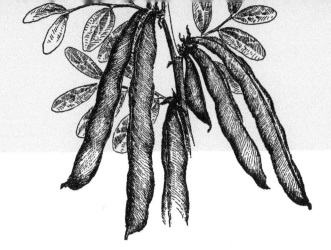

I'm not sure whether it was the copious amounts of beet juice I drank, which increases blood flow, or the countless miles I ran during training, but I ran the 2010 Philadelphia Marathon in 3 hours, 40 minutes, which qualified me for the Boston Marathon. I felt incredibly proud of my athletic feat, but also noticed a vibrancy that hadn't existed before. Gone were the days of antibiotics and inhalers, and I welcomed more natural ways of healing through what I put on (or left off) my plate.

In my clinical and private work as a dietitian today, I aim to mix my Western medical nutrition training with Eastern philosophies and share my belief that food can be incredibly healing. I truly believe that although there is no one-size-fits-all solution when it comes to nutrition, everyone can benefit from more plants in their diet.

If you're seeking ways to improve your overall health and become more familiar with the nutritional value of plant-based foods, this book is for you! I profile 50 nutritional sources that contain powerful healing properties, walk you through how they function, and highlight how to integrate them into your daily life. I hope this book will inspire you to start exploring your own relationship with plant-based nutrition and healing. Lace up your shoes and let me guide you to a healthier and happier you—naturally!

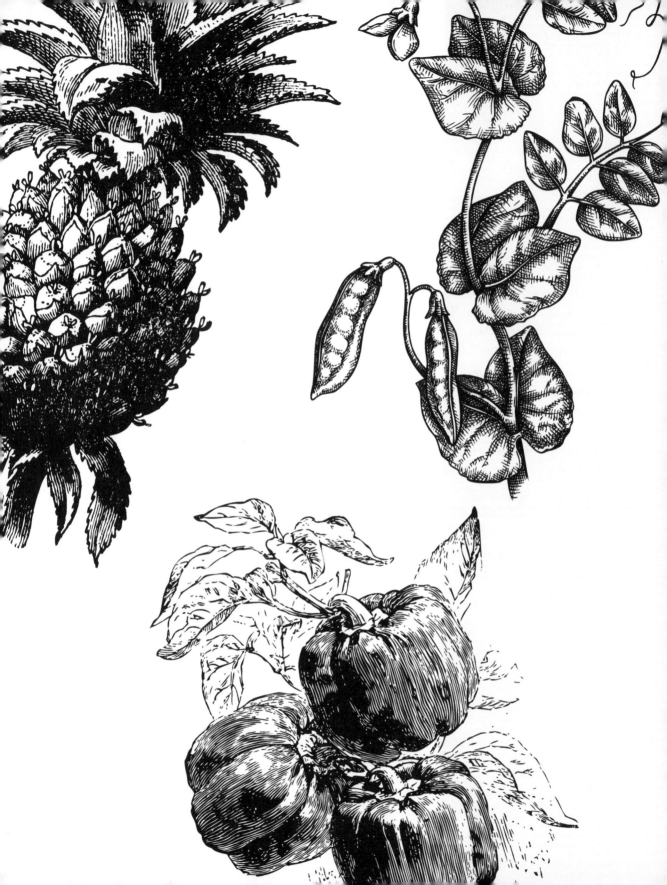

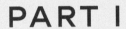

PART I

Food as Medicine

Food has many functions. It can be a source of fuel, a means of celebration, a way to promote growth and survival, and, of course, medicine. People turn to natural sources of healing for various reasons. Perhaps they have chronic conditions they're struggling to manage through traditional medical treatment, or maybe they're interested in preventing common problems associated with poor nutrition, such as diabetes, hypertension, and heart disease. As a dietitian, I aim to share the power of the overall diet for wellness. I frequently "prescribe" specific foods to include or exclude in my clients' daily lives, noting that each food serves a purpose and can be used to promote optimal health. In my opinion, a healthy diet is the most powerful tool you have for protecting your health! Food can affect how you feel physically, and control how genes are expressed, affecting everything from your brain and heart to your energy, hormones, and mood. Whether or not you are seeking to prevent or manage a particular condition, you can use food to be your best, healthiest, and happiest self.

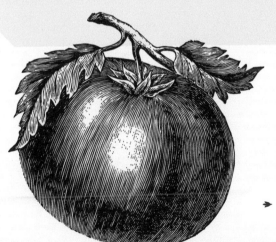

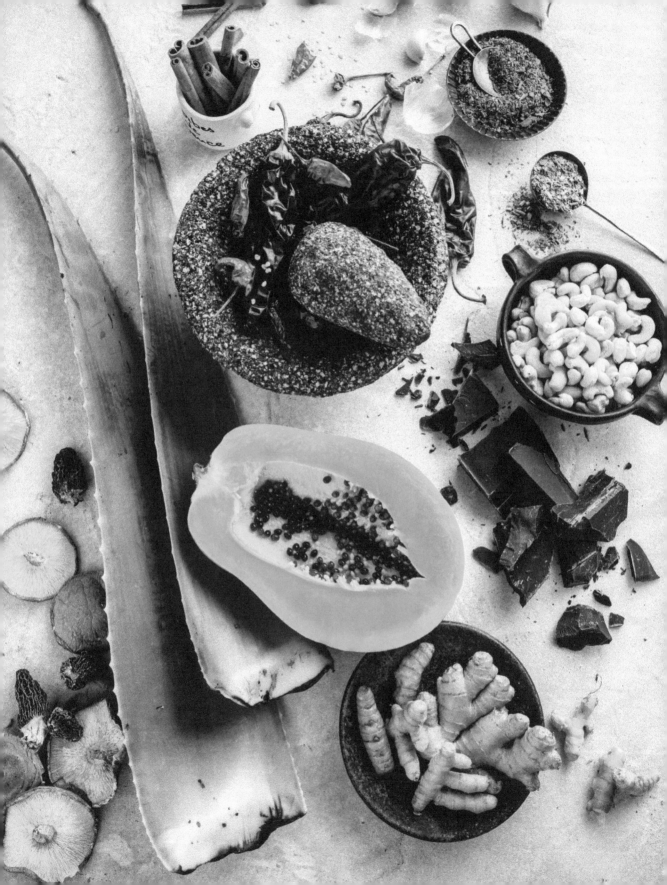

1

History of Nutritional Healing

Plant-based food remedies have been used to prevent and treat diseases since the beginning of humankind. The medicinal properties of food have been used in various cultures and are steeped in cultural beliefs and value systems. Food remedies have trickled down through generations and spread across the globe. We continue to integrate many of these natural remedies into our lives today!

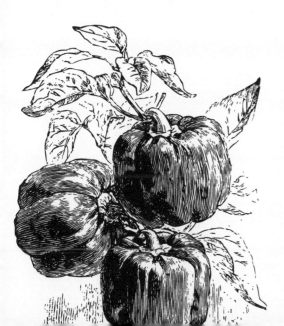

NATURAL REMEDIES AROUND THE WORLD

Fruits and Vegetables

Natural remedies made from plants, such as herbs, spices, fruits, and vegetables, are used across the globe to treat everyday ailments. Plants native to each continent have provided cultures with powerful healing solutions for everything from constipation to colds. Check out the following examples from each continent.

North America

In the United States, "An apple a day keeps the doctor away" is a favorite saying—and it's true! High in fiber, apples have been used to promote digestive health and treat constipation. Cranberries have been used to treat and prevent urinary tract infections. Maple syrup, usually found in Canada and northern US states, is used to fight bacteria internally and externally. Mexico is known for chile peppers, which contain the powerful and warming ingredient, capsaicin. The Maya used chiles to treat asthma and coughs; Aztecs used them to treat

toothaches. The dried, ground form of chile peppers, cayenne pepper, stimulates digestion. Cayenne can be used topically for pain relief or as a gargle to treat sore throats.

South America

South America is home to many plant-based food remedies, including tubers such as potato and yacon. The Incas in Peru were the first to cultivate potatoes, and they used the starchy tuber to treat injuries. One of the most widely studied food remedies is cacao, or chocolate. Mesoamerican communities used cacao to treat everything from indigestion to gout and dysentery. It was also used as a stimulant or treatment for fatigue. In Brazil, cashew nuts are used for gastrointestinal ailments such as stomach ulcers and gastritis. Because of their antioxidant content, cashews are also widely used in the cosmetic industry. In Mayan herbal medicine, papaya was used as a digestive aid. The fruit contains an enzyme, papain, which helps digest proteins and it is used commercially as a red meat tenderizer and for brewing beer. Papain is also used for treating warts and scars.

Africa

Aloe vera, a popular medicinal plant native to North Africa, is used to treat burns. The nutritious aloe vera juice is used to treat heartburn and constipation. Okra is commonly used in African medicine to treat gastritis because the mucilage is thought to lubricate the intestines. Like aloe vera, the okra's mucilage is used topically to heal burns and wounds. Interestingly, the seeds of okra are also toasted, ground, and used as a coffee substitute. Moringa is an incredibly versatile plant that grows quickly and produces leaves even during periods of drought. The leaves have been used to support the high protein, vitamin, and mineral needs of pregnant and nursing mothers. In addition, moringa seeds can be used to purify drinking water.

Asia

Traditional Chinese medicine (TCM) and Ayurveda have demonstrated the use of plant-based remedies for centuries. Asian diets are rich in white rice, which has traditionally been used as a cure for diarrhea. Kimchi, a Korean staple made of salted and fermented vegetables such as cabbage, was historically a way to preserve vegetables before the times of refrigeration. Today, kimchi is widely available and touted as a rich source of probiotics, which can promote optimal digestion. Green tea has been used by TCM practitioners for centuries to relieve

headaches and promote alertness. Now, green tea is widely consumed for its cancer-protective antioxidant capacity and metabolism-boosting qualities. Green tea is also used topically to improve the complexion and boost skin health. Medicinal mushrooms, such as reishi, shiitake, and maitake, have been used for centuries to boost immunity, fight cancer, and improve digestion.

Australia and Oceania

Manuka honey from New Zealand is one of the most well-known (and sweetest) natural healing agents. It is used to treat allergies and external woes such as acne and wounds. Aboriginal people in Australia use the Kakadu plum for its soothing properties. This plum has one of the highest concentrations of vitamin C from any natural source—even more than oranges! Because of its low glycemic index, taro is a desirable tuber for helping modulate blood sugar. The leaves of the taro plant were historically used by Aboriginal people to treat snake and insect bites.

Herbs and Spices

Just like fruits and vegetables, herbs and spices have been used for their medicinal benefits for centuries. Before pharmaceutical drugs were invented, people turned to herbal remedies to treat everything from coughs to rashes and indigestion.

North America

Echinacea is a well-known North American plant with roots and leaves that have been used to strengthen the immune system. It has been shown to reduce the odds of developing a cold and can be effective in reducing the duration of cold and flu symptoms. In the nineteenth century, it was referred to as Indian snakeroot and was used to treat snakebites. Cinnamon originates from India and Sri Lanka but has been widely used in Mexican culture to treat upset stomach, heartburn, and indigestion. Cinnamon has also been used to promote heart health and circulation. Today, cinnamon is used to help stabilize blood sugar levels.

South America

Maca, a native South American root, is a beloved staple medicinal food of the Andean culture. It was used to help support immune function and treat hormonal disorders. Maca is now touted as an effective energy booster and powerful tool for increasing libido and fertility. Indigenous people in South America used yerba mate as a diuretic and stimulating medicinal drink. The tea is now marketed as a weight loss tea that may reduce appetite and help reduce belly fat.

Africa

Teas, including rooibos and chamomile, have been used for centuries for healing and soothing. The South African varietal rooibos was traditionally used as a sleep aid and treatment for headaches. This tea is now widely used as a caffeine-free alternative to black tea with a high antioxidant capacity that may protect against cancer and heart disease. The use of chamomile tea dates back to ancient Egypt, where it was prescribed as a cold remedy. Today it is used as a calming tonic for sleep and anxiety.

Asia

In Asia, herbs and spices have been celebrated for their therapeutic powers for centuries. Ginger was historically used in Japan to treat a cold. It is now used across the globe to relieve nausea and indigestion. In China, garlic is part of the daily diet to prevent and treat respiratory and digestive ailments. It is also a key herb in Ayurvedic medicine, used for its detoxifying properties. Turmeric is best known for its bright yellow color. Used widely in Chinese and Indian medicine, turmeric was traditionally used as a treatment for jaundice and other liver-related diseases. New research shows that turmeric is a powerful anti-inflammatory agent and can be used to prevent cancer and autoimmune diseases.

Australia and Oceania

In Australia, tea tree oil was used by Aboriginal communities as a natural antiseptic for burns and skin infections. It can also be used to treat acne and athlete's foot. Eucalyptus is another Aboriginal remedy traditionally used to relieve coughs, colds, and sore throat. It can also be used topically as a chest rub to provide relief of respiratory infections or to relieve joint pain.

A NOTE OF CAUTION ABOUT HERBAL AND NATURAL REMEDIES

Always consider health concerns when contemplating the use of natural, plant-based, or herbal remedies. Treatments and medications derived from fruits, vegetables, herbs, and spices may cause side effects or interact with medications, with dangerous consequences. The amount you consume, or dosage, of particular natural remedies must also be taken into consideration, as there is a risk of overdose. Note that herbal and "natural" supplements are not subjected to the same strict regulations as traditional pharmaceuticals. Regulations ensure supplements meet specific manufacturing standards, but there is no guarantee they are safe or effective. Please consult with a medical professional prior to using any natural remedies, especially if you take prescription or over-the-counter medication, are pregnant or breastfeeding, or have a chronic health problem. Always choose a reliable source. Independent testing services such as ConsumerLab or Labdoor are helpful resources for finding safe and effective supplements.

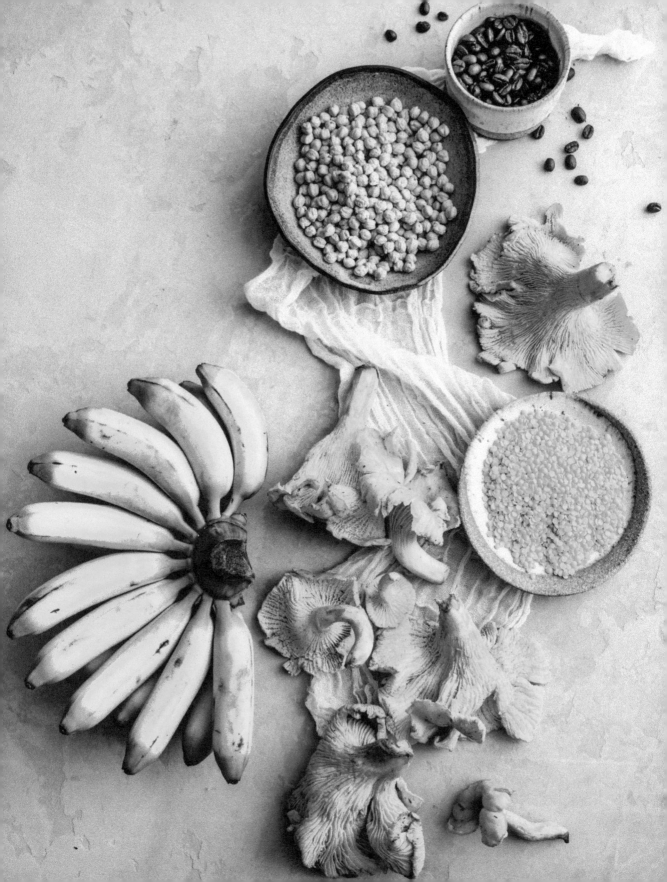

2

Plant Nutrition Basics

We all know we should eat more fruits and vegetables, but do you know why? A plant-based diet full of whole foods eliminates highly refined foods, animal products, and added sugars in favor of minimally processed plant foods, such as vegetables, fruits, whole grains, legumes, nuts, and seeds. This way of eating increases the overall nutritional value of our diet, providing adequate levels of micro- and macronutrients critical for vitality and overall health. A plant-based diet centered on fruits and vegetables has been linked to numerous health benefits, including reduced risks of heart disease, cancer, obesity, and diabetes. In the simplest terms, you are what you eat, and if you consume nutrient-void foods, you'll likely feel that way, too! Consuming a plant-based diet, or just adding more plant-based foods to your current routine, is one of the best tools you have for optimal health.

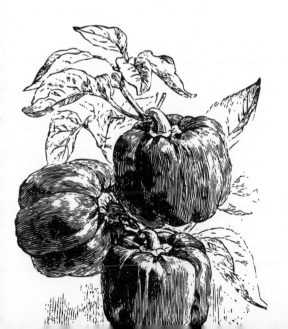

NUTRITIONAL GAPS

Nutrient deficiencies from poor dietary habits can be linked to almost all modern health conditions. You may think of diabetes and heart disease as the heaviest hitters, but cancer, allergies, and autoimmune issues are also huge concerns. Interest in the field of nutrigenomics, or the study of how food influences gene expression and contributes to the prevention, promotion, or treatment of disease, has grown tremendously over the past few years in an effort to try to address, eliminate, and prevent nutrition-related health epidemics.

Ironically, we have an abundant food supply, but we are incredibly malnourished. The standard American (or Western) diet is full of nutritional gaps, or variances between what the body needs and what is consumed to fill those needs. Nutritional gaps can lead to nutrient deficiencies and, eventually, disease. With a diet high in meat, fats and oils, and sugars and sweeteners, and low in plant-based foods, it makes sense that unhealthy eating habits are one of the leading causes of death in the United States.

According to the United States Centers for Disease Control, nutritional deficiencies in the vitamins B_6 and D and the mineral iron are the most prevalent in the United States. These common deficiencies could be eliminated by consuming fruits and vegetables you can find in almost any grocery store. Vitamin B_6, which is critical for normal brain development and nervous system health, is found in chickpeas, bananas, and potatoes. Sunshine and mushrooms are great sources of vitamin D, a nutrient needed for bone health. Iron deficiency can lead to anemia and other health issues, such as decreased cognitive and immune function. Plant-based food sources of iron include lentils, spinach, and cashews. Other nutrients of concern are vitamins C and B_{12} and dietary fiber. A plant-based diet is a simple solution to improving these deficiencies—and a delicious way to bridge the gap!

TOXINS

Environmental toxins, both naturally occurring and made by humans, pose a threat to our health. Naturally occurring heavy metals, such as lead and mercury, and manufactured chemicals, such as BPA-containing plastics and pesticides, can cause cancer, disrupt hormone function, and lead to disease. In the body, these toxins form free radicals, or unstable molecules that damage cells. Free radicals accumulate over time, leading to a state called oxidative stress. Chronic oxidative stress can lead to disease.

Exposure to toxic metals, smoke, and chemicals creates obvious concerns, but many people fail to recognize how everyday products—such as plastic containers, cosmetics, and the food you put on your plate—can affect your toxic load. Although it is impossible to eliminate exposure to toxins completely, you can make educated lifestyle choices to help reduce your exposure. Drink clean, filtered water. Swap plastic containers for glass. Use more natural cleaning and cosmetic products. Choose organic foods to cut down significantly on the harmful pesticides you consume.

Eating a plant-based diet rich in antioxidants is also a great way to reduce your exposure to toxins. Antioxidants such as vitamins A and C and beta-carotene defend your cells against toxins. The powerful compounds work by neutralizing free radicals and protecting cells from oxidative stress. Interestingly, beverages such as coffee and tea are the largest source of antioxidants in Western countries, making up about 79 percent of antioxidants in the average diet. Other superfood sources of antioxidants include blueberries, goji berries, and kale.

IS ORGANIC BETTER?

To be honest, yes, organic is best! Food quality is incredibly important, so choosing organic, locally sourced food, whenever possible, is ideal. What's the difference between organic and nonorganic (or conventional) food? Simply, organic food is produced without pesticides and herbicides. The United States Department of Agriculture (USDA) has strict requirements for labeling and producing organic products to ensure these foods are produced without genetically modified organisms (GMOs) or other harmful substances. Organic produce is often fresher because there are fewer preservatives used. And, in my opinion, it just tastes better!

However, organic produce doesn't just taste better; research shows that organic plant-based foods may also be more nutritious. Studies show that some organic varieties of foods contain greater levels of vitamin C, iron, magnesium, and phosphorus than the same nonorganic food. Organics are also higher in antioxidant phytochemicals. If the organic price tag is a deterrent, check out the Environmental Working Group's (EWG) Dirty Dozen™ and Clean Fifteen™ lists. Each year, the EWG ranks the pesticide contamination of 47 popular fruits and vegetables and offers shopping guides for consumers to help them reduce their exposure to toxic chemicals. If you can't buy everything organic, at least try to buy the Dirty Dozen as organic, when you can.

An organic, plant-based diet is not only good for you, it's good for the environment! Sustainable practices, including organic farming, can help fight global warming and environmental decline by reducing greenhouse gases, water consumption, and factory farming.

FOOD PYRAMID EVOLUTION

The USDA published the first model of its Food Pyramid in 1992. This "Eating Right Pyramid" recommended that bread, cereal, rice, and pasta make up the majority of our diet, followed by smaller portions of fruits, vegetables, dairy, meats, and fats. Critics argued that this visual failed to identify the difference between refined and whole grains and promoted the US dairy, beef, and grain industries rather than the health of the general public. In 2005, the "MyPyramid Food Guidance System" introduced a simplified pyramid food pattern. This visual still encouraged a high intake of grains but addressed concepts of moderation and variety of foods, as well as physical activity. The pyramid design was replaced in 2011 by MyPlate, a mealtime visual that recommends including half a plate of fruits and vegetables and making at least half the grains on your plate whole grains. Over time, the suggested servings of fruits and vegetables have increased, and the MyPlate visual encourages Americans to create meals comprising more plant-based foods.

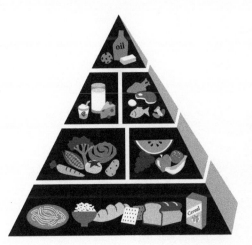

OLD

1992 Food Pyramid

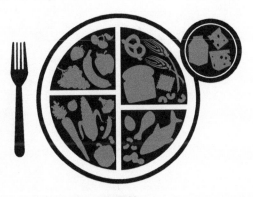

NEW

My Plate

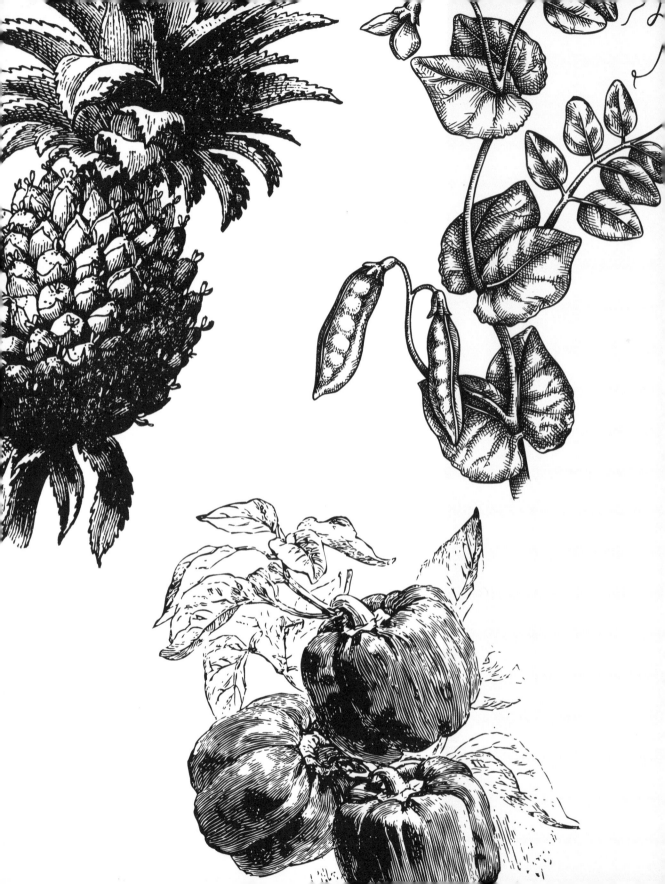

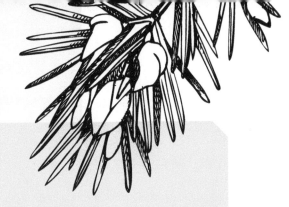

PART II

50 Powerhouse Healing Sources

So, what are these natural healing sources? Let's dive in deeper to learn more about some powerhouse healing sources. No matter what the issue, it's likely a plant-based food may be able to help. This section profiles 50 nutritional sources and their health benefits. Join me as I walk you through how to implement each source into your daily life. I promise that these easy recipes are not only delicious, they're also good for you!

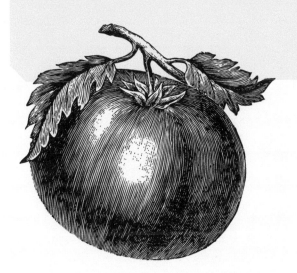

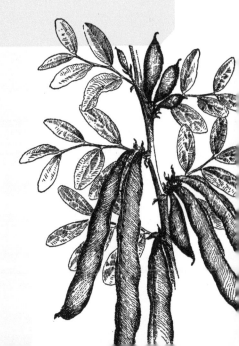

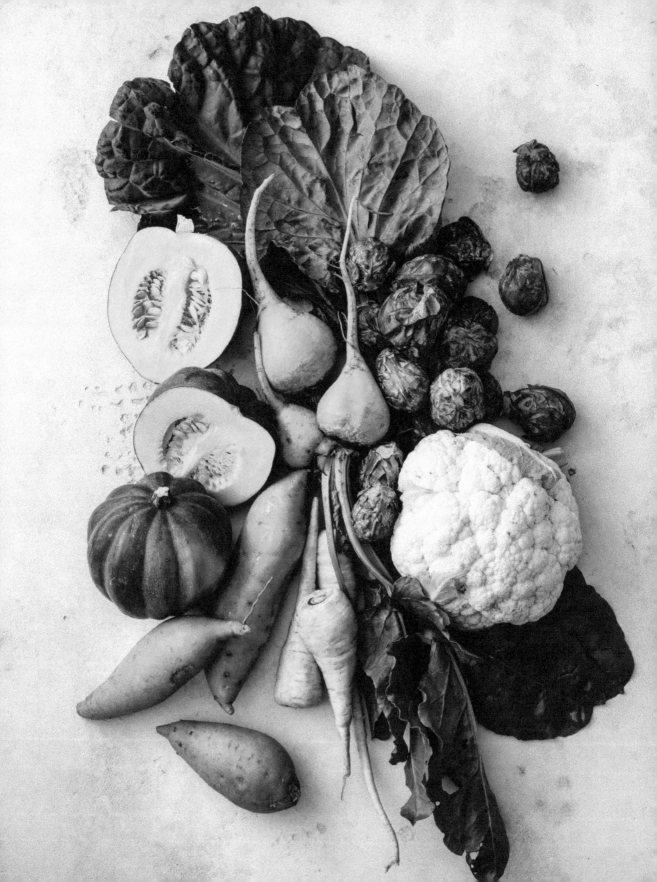

3

Vegetables

Carrots, kale, and parsnips . . . oh my! Let's start with my favorite food group: vegetables. As a dietitian, I recommend vegetables as the basis of a healthy diet. They're full of fiber, vitamins, and minerals and, well, they're delicious. The way you prepare vegetables is key to making them taste great, and as you'll learn, the preparation can even improve their nutritional content. I'm confident I can convert any vegetable naysayer to a veggie lover. If you're already a veg-head, fabulous! Let's explore how to use these incredible foods to boost your health.

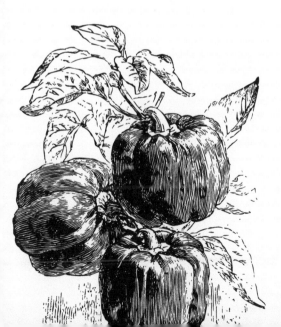

SWEET POTATOES

Sweet potatoes are a great source of free radical–fighting antioxidants, especially the carotenoids lutein and zeaxanthin. These two carotenoids are very beneficial to eye health, filtering light, and helping maintain vision. Although sweet potatoes live up to their name, they don't raise blood sugar as much as the russet potato. Sweet potatoes were historically used to promote optimal digestion and help nursing moms produce breastmilk. They can be used topically to soothe skin and protect against aging.

AT A GLANCE: beta-carotene, lutein, vitamins C and E, and zeaxanthin

HEALING POWER: Sweet potatoes are packed with filling fiber and powerful antioxidants, including vitamins C and E. Beta-carotene, the antioxidant responsible for the bright red-orange pigment of the flesh, is a precursor to vitamin A. Beta-carotene works in tandem with vitamins C and E to fight inflammation by neutralizing free radicals in the body. The complex carbohydrate and fiber content of sweet potatoes works to ease digestion and promote weight maintenance. The complex carbohydrates are broken down more slowly than simple carbohydrates, and insoluble and soluble fiber helps bulk stool and move the waste material through the digestive system. For the highest fiber content, keep the skin on!

HEALTH BENEFITS/MEDICAL CONDITIONS: Sweet potatoes may help promote blood sugar control in people with diabetes, as the natural fiber slows the uptake of carbohydrates in the body, modulating the response of blood sugar and preventing a large spike. The high fiber content may also benefit those seeking to lose weight. Fiber helps fill the stomach and sustain energy for long periods, so you won't be hungry for hours after eating. The antioxidants in sweet potatoes help fight free radicals that can lead to cancer and heart disease and protect vision.

CONSUMPTION: 1 cup, or about 1 medium sweet potato

SPICY BAKED SWEET POTATO FRIES

Serves 4

Prep time: 10 minutes

Cook time: 30 minutes

These "healthier for you" fries are a great vitamin C–rich side dish or snack. When you heat sweet potatoes, the starch is broken down into a sugar called maltose. This maltose isn't as sweet as typical table sugar, but it lends a rich taste that is complemented by savory garlic and spicy red pepper flakes. If you love sweet potatoes, but are not into spice, check out the Variation Tip.

INGREDIENTS

2 or 3 medium sweet potatoes, cut into ¼-inch-thick fry-shaped pieces

2 tablespoons extra-virgin olive oil

½ teaspoon sea salt

½ teaspoon garlic powder

½ teaspoon red pepper flakes

½ teaspoon freshly ground black pepper

VARIATION TIP

If you want more spice, increase the red pepper flakes to 1 teaspoon or add ½ teaspoon cayenne pepper. If you don't like spicy foods, omit the red pepper flakes, or swap them for ½ teaspoon onion powder.

1. Preheat the oven to 450°F. Line a large rimmed sheet pan with parchment paper.

2. In a large bowl, toss together the sweet potato fries, olive oil, salt, garlic powder, red pepper flakes, and black pepper to coat. Arrange the fries in a single layer on the prepared sheet pan, being sure not to overcrowd them. If needed, use an additional baking sheet.

3. Bake for 25 to 30 minutes, turning the fries over with a spatula halfway through the baking time. When the fries are golden and baked to your desired crispness, remove from the oven and serve warm.

STORAGE TIP

These fries keep for about 4 days in the refrigerator.

Per Serving: Calories: 146; Saturated Fat: 1g; Total Fat: 7g; Protein: 2g; Total Carbs: 20g; Fiber: 3g; Sodium: 288mg

BLACK BEAN–STUFFED SWEET POTATO

Serves 1

Prep time: 10 minutes

This quick meal is full of protein, fiber-rich carbohydrates, and healthy fat, which will help keep you satisfied for a long time. Combining all three macronutrients helps make a fully balanced meal, which sustains energy and keeps blood sugar levels stable.

INGREDIENTS

1 medium sweet potato, cooked and halved lengthwise

1 cup cooked black beans

½ teaspoon ground cumin

⅛ teaspoon smoked paprika

½ avocado, peeled, pitted, and cut into slices

2 tablespoons salsa

COOKING TIP

To bake a sweet potato, using a fork, pierce a few holes in the skin. If using the microwave, wet a paper towel and squeeze out the excess water. Wrap the sweet potato in the towel, then place it on a microwave-safe plate. Microwave on high power for 5 minutes, then carefully turn the potato over and cook for another 3 to 5 minutes, or until the sweet potato is fully cooked. To bake in the oven, tightly wrap the potato in aluminum foil. Place the potato on a baking sheet and bake at 400°F for 30 to 45 minutes, or until soft.

1. Scoop the flesh from each half of the sweet potato into a small bowl, leaving enough flesh intact on the skin to maintain the shape of the potato shells. Using a fork, mash the sweet potato flesh.

2. Add the black beans, cumin, and paprika to the mashed flesh. Stir to combine well. Scoop the mixture back into the sweet potato skins.

3. Top each half with sliced avocado and 1 tablespoon salsa.

INGREDIENT TIP

Cook the black beans yourself or use canned. If using canned beans, choose a no-salt-added variety, rinse them well, and heat them before adding to the sweet potato mash.

Per Serving: Calories: 496; Saturated Fat: 2g; Total Fat: 15g; Protein: 20g; Total Carbs: 77g; Fiber: 25g; Sodium: 274mg

BEETS

The natural plant pigment betalain is responsible for the vibrant red color of beets. Beets come in many varieties, including yellow, white, pink, and, my favorite, candy cane. Although current research has highlighted beet juice as an athletic performance enhancer, beets have been used in traditional Chinese medicine and Ayurveda for centuries to treat conditions related to circulation, anemia, and the heart. Beets were thought to purify the blood, promote menstruation, and improve liver function. Their bright red juice is used as a food dye and the sweet sugars are used to make sugar. Don't forget the beet greens! They are incredibly nutritious and can be sautéed or steamed like spinach.

AT A GLANCE: folate, iron, potassium

HEALING POWER: The high folic acid and iron content of beets builds and sustains blood supply. Folic acid is a vitamin that helps the body break down protein, make new cells, and produce DNA. Iron is a mineral that helps produce red blood cells and that is found primarily in hemoglobin, which transfers oxygen in the blood from the lungs to necessary tissues. Beets supply your body with these necessary nutrients, as well as potassium, which promotes normal blood pressure and fluid balance. Beets are also rich in chemicals called nitrates, which the body changes into nitric oxide. Nitric oxide promotes vasodilation, or relaxation of the inner muscles of the blood vessels, which improves circulation.

HEALTH BENEFITS/MEDICAL CONDITIONS: The nitric oxide and potassium in beets can help reduce blood pressure and promote heart health. The high content of dietary nitrates may boost athletic performance by improving the efficiency of mitochondria. Beet juice may boost stamina, helping you exercise longer. Folate is incredibly important during pregnancy and can help prevent neural tube defects in the baby. The fiber content in beets can be beneficial for weight loss and digestion. Dietary fiber moves slowly through the digestive tract, helping promote satiety, which, in turn, supports weight loss. This fiber adds bulk to stool, improving digestive health and fighting constipation.

CONSUMPTION: 1 cup cooked or raw beets

ROASTED BEET HUMMUS

Serves 4

Prep time: 10 minutes

This nutrient-dense dish offers a flavorful alternative to traditional hummus and boosts the fiber, folate, and vitamin C content. The creamy blend pairs perfectly with high-fiber crackers, whole-wheat pita, cucumber slices, or carrots! Roast the beet yourself or use canned beets for a quicker option.

INGREDIENTS

1 (15-ounce) can no-salt-added chickpeas, drained and rinsed

1 beet, roasted, peeled, and coarsely chopped

3 tablespoons tahini

2 garlic cloves, peeled

Juice of ½ large lemon, plus more as needed

1 teaspoon salt, plus more as needed

1 teaspoon freshly ground black pepper, plus more as needed

¼ cup extra-virgin olive oil

1. In a food processor, combine the chickpeas, beet, tahini, garlic, lemon juice, salt, and pepper and blend until smooth.

2. While the blender is running, slowly drizzle in the olive oil.

3. Taste and season with more salt, pepper, or lemon juice, as needed. Add a bit of water if the consistency is too thick.

STORAGE TIP

This hummus can be refrigerated in an airtight container for up to 1 week.

COOKING TIP

To roast a beet, remove the stem and roots and scrub the beet well. Preheat the oven to 375°F. Place the beet on a large sheet of aluminum foil, drizzle it with a bit of avocado oil or olive oil, and tightly wrap it. Roast for 1 hour in the oven. Cool, then peel (or retain the skin if you want more fiber).

Per Serving: Calories: 292; Saturated Fat: 3g; Total Fat: 20g; Protein: 8g; Total Carbs: 23g; Fiber: 6g; Sodium: 620mg

CACAO BEET SMOOTHIE

Serves 2

Prep time: 5 minutes

This beautiful red blend offers a sweeter variation of a typical beet dish. Betalain, the natural plant pigment responsible for beets' vibrant red color, provides powerful antioxidant and anti-inflammatory powers. The combination of the cacao and the beets packs vitamins, minerals, antioxidants, and fiber into a sippable smoothie powerhouse.

INGREDIENTS

1 cup unsweetened plain almond milk

1 beet, roasted, peeled, and coarsely chopped

½ banana, peeled and frozen

½ cup frozen spinach

4 frozen strawberries

2 tablespoons nondairy plain yogurt (coconut, almond, cashew, etc.)

2 tablespoons cacao powder

½ teaspoon vanilla extract

½ teaspoon ground cinnamon

3 or 4 ice cubes

In a high-speed blender, combine the almond milk, beet, banana, spinach, strawberries, yogurt, cacao powder, vanilla, cinnamon, and ice. Blend on high speed until smooth.

VARIATION TIP

Top with 1 tablespoon cacao nibs for some crunch and an extra dose of muscle-relaxing magnesium.

COOKING TIP

If you choose to roast your own beets, try using a slow cooker. Trim and wash the beets, then put them in a slow cooker with ¼ cup water. Cover the cooker and cook on high heat for 4 hours. Once beets are cooked and cooled, peel and refrigerate until needed.

Per Serving: Calories: 170; Saturated Fat: 3g; Total Fat: 8g; Protein: 7g; Total Carbs: 28g; Fiber: 10g; Sodium: 225mg

CARROTS

Carrots are one of the best sources of the antioxidant beta-carotene. In Asian tradition, carrots are believed to be an alkaline-forming food and are used to treat acidic issues such as acne and tonsillitis. You've likely heard of turning orange from eating too many carrots, or the condition called carotenoderma. Although adding carrots to your daily routine is great for many reasons, as with all foods, they should be consumed in moderation!

AT A GLANCE: beta-carotene, biotin, vitamin K

HEALING POWER: The high beta-carotene content in carrots converts to vitamin A in the body. Vitamin A, in turn, promotes good vision and eye health by forming a pigment called rhodopsin, which increases your ability to see in dim light. Carrots contain another free radical–fighting carotenoid, alpha-carotene. This carotenoid works as an antioxidant and has anticarcinogenic powers. Carrots are a biotin-rich food, and biotin is necessary for cell signaling and helps the body metabolize food. Vitamin K works in tandem with calcium to promote optimal bone health.

HEALTH BENEFITS/MEDICAL CONDITIONS: Carrots are great for eye health and may help treat people who have trouble with night blindness or night vision. They may also protect against macular degeneration. Carrots, with their high content of carotenoids, may help protect against cancer. Carrots are a high-fiber food and can help promote good digestive health. They're known as a good food for detoxing because of their high antioxidant content. Carrots contain high amounts of biotin, making them great for hair, skin, and nail health. Crunching on carrots may be good for your bones because of high vitamin A and K levels.

CONSUMPTION: 1 cup, raw when possible, or cooked with minimal heat exposure

ROASTED CARROTS WITH CUMIN AND TURMERIC

Serves 6 to 8

Prep time: 10 minutes

Cook time: 40 minutes

Did you know that cooking carrots with the skin on can increase their nutritional benefit? When carrots are cooked, the levels of beta-carotene and phenolic acids are increased. Keeping the skin on the carrot increases not only the fiber, but also the vitamin C and niacin, as they are most concentrated in the peel. Note that boiling carrots may allow water-soluble nutrients (like vitamin C and B vitamins) to leach into the cooking water, which is usually discarded, so either keep the water to use in another recipe, like soup, or try a different cooking method, like roasting or steaming.

INGREDIENTS

¼ cup extra-virgin olive oil

2 garlic cloves, finely minced

1 teaspoon ground cumin

1 teaspoon ground turmeric

2 pounds carrots, halved lengthwise

Salt

Freshly ground black pepper

1. Preheat the oven to 450°F. Line a baking sheet with parchment paper.

2. In a large bowl, whisk the olive oil, garlic, cumin, and turmeric to blend.

3. Toss the carrots in the oil mixture and season with salt and pepper. Transfer the carrots to the prepared baking sheet and spread them into a single layer.

4. Roast for 35 to 40 minutes, turning the carrots every 15 minutes, until the carrots are tender.

VARIATION TIP

You can choose regular carrots or rainbow varieties (purple, yellow, white). Purple carrots, in particular, contain potent antioxidants called anthocyanins, which are found in other purple fruits and veggies like blackberries, cabbage, and grapes. For an extra boost of color, flavor, and nutrition, garnish with some chopped fresh parsley.

Per Serving: Calories: 138; Saturated Fat: 1g; Total Fat: 9g; Protein: 1g; Total Carbs: 16g; Fiber: 4g; Sodium: 132mg

SPIRALIZED LEMON DIJON CARROT SALAD

Serves 3

Prep time: 15 minutes

This vibrant, colorful salad is an easy side dish. Raw carrots provide a satisfying crunch and tons of beta-carotene, fiber, and antioxidants. Beta-carotene is a precursor to the fat-soluble vitamin A. The olive oil in this dish helps increase the absorption of vitamin A in the body, which is made in the intestines from beta-carotene.

INGREDIENTS

1 tablespoon Dijon mustard

1 tablespoon freshly squeezed lemon juice

1 tablespoon extra-virgin olive oil

1 tablespoon finely chopped shallot

¼ teaspoon grated lemon zest

1 pound carrots, peeled and spiralized

Salt

Freshly ground black pepper

1. In a large bowl, whisk the mustard, lemon juice, olive oil, shallot, and lemon zest to blend.

2. Add the carrots to the bowl and toss to combine. Season with salt and pepper.

PREPARATION TIP

If you don't have a spiralizer, use pre-shredded carrots, a regular peeler, or simply cut the carrots into skinny ribbons.

SUBSTITUTION TIP

Use any kind of carrot you like. I recommend a mix of yellow, purple, and typical orange carrots to get a combination of flavors and colors!

Per Serving: Calories: 109; Saturated Fat: 1g; Total Fat: 5g; Protein: 2g; Total Carbs: 16g; Fiber: 4g; Sodium: 215mg

PARSNIPS

Closely related to carrots and parsley, parsnips are a root vegetable with a nutty taste. They're tasty when roasted and can work wonders for the digestive system. Like carrots, they usually come with green leafy tops, which you should snip off before storing the root in the refrigerator. It's best to store parsnips in cold temperatures to prevent them from drying out. Parsnips have been cultivated since ancient times and were used medicinally by the Romans, who believed parsnips to be an aphrodisiac.

AT A GLANCE: fiber, folate, potassium

HEALING POWER: Parsnips are a great vasodilator because of their high potassium content. Potassium helps promote the widening of blood vessels and the relaxation of the smooth muscle of the blood vessels, which allows blood to flow more smoothly. Dietary fiber in parsnips can help reduce cholesterol levels. In the digestive system, the soluble fiber from parsnips attaches to cholesterol and helps eliminate it. This soluble fiber also forms a gel-like consistency that bulks the stool and promotes movement through the digestive tract.

HEALTH BENEFITS/MEDICAL CONDITIONS: Parsnips are great for heart health. The vasodilating potassium and cholesterol-reducing qualities help promote optimal blood flow and reduce stress on the heart. The high dietary fiber content in parsnips is also cardioprotective and promotes good digestion. Soluble fiber in parsnips may protect against diverticulitis. Eating parsnips may also promote weight loss, as the fiber will help you feel fuller longer. Folate is critical for pregnant women, reducing the risk of infant neural tube defects.

CONSUMPTION: 1 cup cooked

CARROT PARSNIP SOUP WITH CHIVES AND PUMPKIN SEEDS

Serves 4

Prep time: 20 minutes

Cook time: 30 minutes

Carrots and parsnips are high in nutrients and low in calories. They are rich sources of soluble and insoluble fiber, which help boost gut health and keep you feeling fuller longer. Topping this soup with pumpkin seeds increases satiating protein and healthy fat content!

INGREDIENTS

1½ pounds carrots, peeled, halved lengthwise, and cut into ½-inch pieces

1 pound parsnips, peeled, halved lengthwise, and cut into ½-inch pieces

1 yellow onion, roughly chopped

3 garlic cloves, finely minced

¼ cup extra-virgin olive oil

Salt

Freshly ground black pepper

4 cups low-sodium vegetable broth, divided

½ cup pumpkin seeds

¼ cup finely chopped fresh chives

1. Preheat the oven to 450°F. Line two baking sheets with parchment paper.

2. In a large bowl, toss together the carrots, parsnips, onion, garlic, and olive oil to coat the vegetables. Season well with salt and pepper. Transfer the vegetables to the prepared baking sheets and spread them into a single layer.

3. Roast for about 30 minutes, or until the vegetables are cooked through.

4. In a blender, working in batches, combine half the roasted vegetables with 2 cups of vegetable broth. Purée until smooth. Add water to thin, as needed. Repeat with the remaining vegetables and broth.

5. Mix the batches of blended soup, taste, and adjust the seasoning.

6. Serve each bowl topped with 2 tablespoons of pumpkin seeds and 1 tablespoon of chives.

STORAGE TIP

Freeze leftover soup for up to 4 months.

Per Serving: Calories: 386; Saturated Fat: 3g; Total Fat: 21g; Protein: 10g; Total Carbs: 45g; Fiber: 11g; Sodium: 242mg

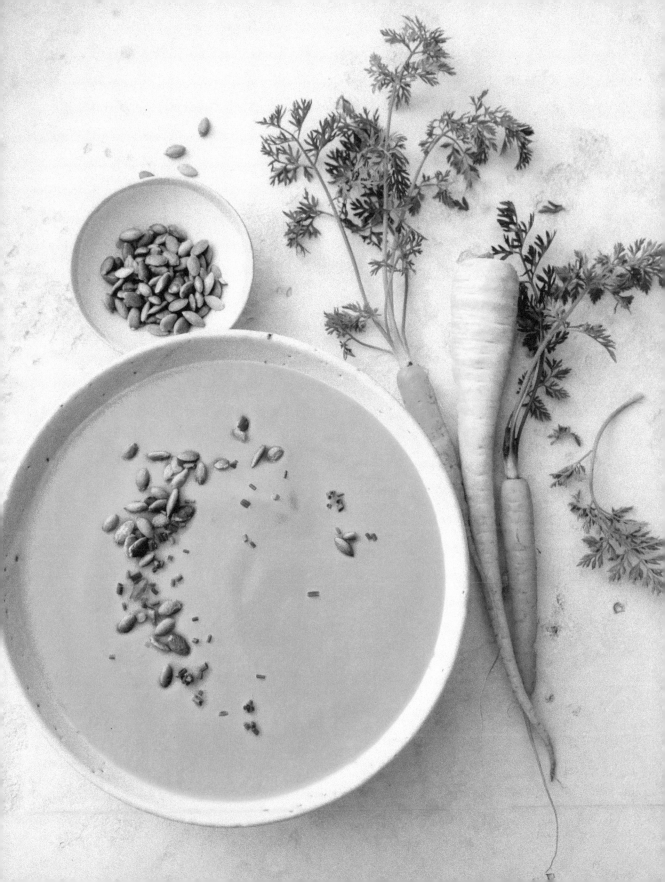

ROSEMARY PARSNIP FRIES

Serves 6
Prep time: 10 minutes
Cook time: 20 minutes

Closely related to carrots and other root vegetables, parsnips have a sweet, slightly nutty flavor that pairs well with strong herbs such as rosemary. Because of their high fiber content (both soluble and insoluble), parsnips can help improve digestive health, regulate blood sugar levels, and enhance heart health.

INGREDIENTS

¼ cup extra-virgin olive oil

1 tablespoon finely chopped fresh rosemary leaves, or 1 teaspoon dried rosemary

1 garlic clove, finely minced

2 pounds parsnips, cut into ½-inch-thick fry shapes

Salt

Freshly ground black pepper

1. Preheat the oven to 450°F.

2. In a small bowl, whisk the olive oil, rosemary, and garlic to combine.

3. Place the parsnips on a large rimmed baking sheet and pour the olive oil mixture over the parsnips. Toss to coat. Spread the parsnips into a single layer. Season with salt and pepper.

4. Bake for 20 minutes, turning the fries over with a spatula halfway through the baking time. When the parsnips are tender and slightly browned, remove them from the oven and serve warm.

VARIATION TIP

Parsnips are also great in chip form! Use a mandoline or sharp knife to cut the parsnips into small, thin slices, and follow steps 2 and 3 above. Bake for 25 to 35 minutes, or until brown and crispy. You may need additional baking sheets.

Per Serving: Calories: 187; Saturated Fat: 1g; Total Fat: 9g; Protein: 2g; Total Carbs: 28g; Fiber: 8g; Sodium: 42mg

CUCUMBERS

Cucumbers are incredibly hydrating and offer a wide array of internal and external health benefits. Topically (i.e., used on the skin), cucumbers can reduce puffiness around the eyes and make you look refreshed. Internally, they help reduce inflammation. They provide a natural cooling effect and supply powerful antioxidants to slow aging. Cucumbers have long been used as a laxative and diuretic, but the term "cool as a cucumber" came about when seventeenth-century physicians prescribed cucumbers for cooling a fever.

AT A GLANCE: cucurbitacin, lignan, magnesium

HEALING POWER: Cucumbers are mostly made up of water and are an incredible diuretic. They help flush water through the body and reduce inflammation, which decreases swelling. The high water content of cucumbers promotes optimal hydration in the body, which can boost metabolism, improve energy, and even boost the immune system. Cucumbers are thought to have an alkalizing affect. They help balance the acid in our bodies that comes from consuming things such as processed foods and caffeine. Cucumbers are rich in magnesium, which relaxes muscles to promote good circulation and optimal digestion. Cucumbers contain large amounts of phytonutrients, including cucurbitacins and lignans, with anticancer benefits. Cucurbitacins have a high amount of anti-inflammatory potential and may inhibit tumor growth. Lignans work in conjunction with bacteria in the digestive tract. They bind to certain receptors and are converted into cancer-protective nutrients.

HEALTH BENEFITS/MEDICAL CONDITIONS: The high water and low calorie content in cucumbers makes them a great food for weight loss. You can eat a large volume (low calories) and feel more satiated (high water content) for longer. Cucumbers also act as a natural diuretic and can be used to fight bloat. Pickles are a form of fermented cucumber, which can be a good source of beneficial bacteria, or probiotics (some people may need to watch the sodium content though). The magnesium content in cucumbers, coupled with the water content, can help fight constipation. Magnesium helps promote optimal heart health. The cucurbitacin and lignan content helps protect against cancer.

CONSUMPTION: ½ cup sliced cucumber

CHOPPED GREEK SALAD PITA

Serves 2

Prep time: 15 minutes

This savory chopped Greek salad is incredibly hydrating and offers a satisfying crunch. Consuming water-rich vegetables, such as tomatoes, cucumbers, and peppers, helps increase overall hydration levels in the body. Being adequately hydrated is beneficial to almost all systems: It helps muscles and joints stay lubricated, keeps skin supple, and fights fatigue.

INGREDIENTS

¼ cup extra-virgin olive oil

3 tablespoons red wine vinegar

2 teaspoons dried oregano

1 teaspoon honey

1 pint cherry tomatoes, halved

1 medium cucumber, seeded and chopped

1 red bell pepper, chopped

½ medium red onion, chopped

½ cup pitted Kalamata olives

2 whole-wheat pitas, halved and warmed

1. In a small bowl, whisk the olive oil, vinegar, oregano, and honey to blend.

2. In a large bowl, gently stir together the tomatoes, cucumber, red bell pepper, red onion, and olives. Drizzle the dressing over the salad and mix well to combine.

3. Serve each salad in a warmed pita.

VARIATION TIP

To make the salad vegan, skip the honey, or use maple syrup instead. If you want to increase the protein content, add 1 cup cooked chickpeas.

Per Serving: Calories: 530; Saturated Fat: 5g; Total Fat: 31g; Protein: 10g; Total Carbs: 61g; Fiber: 11g; Sodium: 649mg

SIMPLE CUCUMBER SALAD

Serves 2

Prep time: 5 minutes

This simple Asian-inspired cucumber salad is one of my favorite dishes. Sesame seeds are a great source of nondairy calcium, B vitamins, and protein. The combination of cucumbers and sesame seeds equals a nutritious and tasty snack.

INGREDIENTS

3 tablespoons rice wine vinegar

1 teaspoon honey

1 teaspoon sesame oil

1 teaspoon flaky white sea salt

½ teaspoon freshly ground black pepper

2 English cucumbers, peeled, seeded, and thinly sliced

¼ cup thinly sliced red onion

1 tablespoon sesame seeds

Red pepper flakes, for garnish (optional)

1. In a small bowl, whisk the vinegar, honey, sesame oil, salt, and pepper to combine.

2. In a large bowl, combine the cucumbers and red onion. Add the dressing and toss to coat the cucumbers and onion.

3. Serve garnished with sesame seeds and red pepper flakes (if using).

SUBSTITUTION TIP

No need to use the honey or sesame oil if you don't want to. The rice wine vinegar by itself contributes a ton of flavor.

Per Serving: Calories: 124; Saturated Fat: 1g; Total Fat: 5g; Protein: 3g; Total Carbs: 17g; Fiber: 3g; Sodium: 202mg

FENNEL

Traditionally used by the Greeks and Romans as medicine and insect repellent, fennel was highly regarded in ancient times. It is believed that fennel tea was given to ancient warriors to provide courage before battle. In traditional Chinese medicine, fennel seeds are regarded as a warming food, and can be used along with other seeds, such as flaxseed and fenugreek, to treat asthma. Typically used in Mediterranean and Italian dishes, the anise-flavored vegetable and its seeds are highly nutritious and healing.

AT A GLANCE: anethole, fiber, potassium, vitamin C

HEALING POWER: The vitamin C in fennel offers antioxidant protection and immune support. This water-soluble vitamin helps reverse and prevent the damage of free radicals in the body. Fennel contains many other phytonutrients with antioxidant effects. The most interesting of these phytonutrients is anethole. Anethole is the compound that contributes the anise flavor and it works in the body to block inflammation and carcinogenesis. Although the particular mechanism is unknown, researchers believe that anethole interferes with the signaling process of certain gene expressions, suppressing inflammation and preventing carcinogenesis. The important mineral potassium functions much like an electrolyte in the body, helping regulate fluid balance, muscle contractions, and nerve signaling. Potassium is key for optimal cardiac health.

Fennel seed is an incredible digestive aid and is used to calm the stomach, reducing spasms, gas, and nausea and preventing cramping.

HEALTH BENEFITS/MEDICAL CONDITIONS: Fennel's high vitamin C content may help fight the common cold and flu. The antioxidant effects of vitamin C and the phytonutrient anethole may help prevent cancer and decrease the amount of inflammation in the body. The high fiber and potassium levels in fennel may help lower blood pressure, reducing the overall risk of stroke and heart attacks. The fiber in fennel helps promote satiety and digestive ease, which may lead to weight loss. Fennel seed, usually in the form of a tea, can be used to reduce symptoms of irritable bowel syndrome, leaky gut, and other digestive disorders.

CONSUMPTION: 1 cup raw, or ½ cup cooked

BRUSSELS SPROUTS WITH FENNEL, APPLE, AND WALNUTS

Serves 6

Prep time: 20 minutes

Cook time: 3 minutes

This tasty raw salad, full of powerful cruciferous Brussels sprouts and phytonutrient-packed fennel, supports detoxification pathways. Eating raw vegetables means you preserve the antioxidant and water-soluble vitamin content that can be lost during cooking. Your immune system will thank you, as Brussels sprouts and fennel are both chock-full of vitamin C.

INGREDIENTS

1 cup walnut halves

¼ cup extra-virgin olive oil

2 tablespoons freshly squeezed lemon juice

1 garlic clove, finely minced

8 ounces Brussels sprouts, shredded or roughly chopped (2 cups)

1 fennel bulb, cored and thinly sliced

1 apple, cored and chopped

Salt

Freshly ground black pepper

1. In a dry skillet over low heat, heat the walnut halves for about 3 minutes, stirring frequently, until evenly toasted. Transfer to a cutting board and roughly chop.

2. In a large bowl, whisk the olive oil, lemon juice, and garlic to combine. Add the Brussels sprouts and toss until they are evenly coated. Let sit for 5 to 10 minutes.

3. Add the fennel, apple, and toasted walnuts. Toss to combine and season with salt and pepper.

INGREDIENT TIP

Cut prep time by using pre-shredded Brussels sprouts. Honeycrisp and Pink Lady are my favorite apple varieties to use in this dish.

VARIATION TIP

If raw vegetables make you feel gassy, try cooking the Brussels sprouts and fennel. Add the olive oil and garlic to the skillet used to toast the walnuts. Sauté the garlic for 1 minute, then add the Brussels sprouts and fennel and sauté until soft. Remove from the heat and stir in the apple and lemon juice.

Per Serving: Calories: 261; Saturated Fat: 3g; Total Fat: 23g; Protein: 5g; Total Carbs: 15g; Fiber: 5g; Sodium: 58mg

ARUGULA AND FENNEL SALAD WITH LEMON AND PINE NUTS

Serves 2

Prep time: 10 minutes

If you're looking for a light, bright, fresh-tasting salad, this one is for you! The peppery flavor of arugula pairs well with the fennel and lemon, which are both great for improving digestion and banishing bloat. The toasted pine nuts add a nutty flavor, as well healthy fat and protein.

INGREDIENTS

2 cups baby arugula

1 fennel bulb, cored and thinly sliced

2 tablespoons extra-virgin olive oil

2 tablespoons freshly squeezed lemon juice

3 tablespoons pine nuts, toasted

Salt

Freshly ground black pepper

1. In a large bowl, toss together the arugula and fennel.

2. Drizzle the vegetables with olive oil and lemon juice and toss well to coat.

3. Sprinkle the pine nuts on top. Season with salt and pepper.

INGREDIENT TIP

Selecting a high-quality olive oil is important. Always purchase organically grown, extra-virgin olive oils. Select oils that come in dark glass bottles and store them in a cool place (away from the stove, but not in the refrigerator) to preserve their phenol levels.

COOKING TIP

To toast the pine nuts: In a dry skillet over medium-low heat, toast the nuts for about 2 minutes until fragrant and lightly browned. Transfer to a plate or bowl to cool.

Per Serving: Calories: 252; Saturated Fat: 3g; Total Fat: 23g; Protein: 4g; Total Carbs: 11g; Fiber: 5g; Sodium: 147mg

SPINACH

Spinach is thought to be one of the healthiest foods of all because of its high antioxidant and nutrient levels. Cooking spinach is quite easy, but don't be shocked when the volume reduces quite drastically. For this reason, cooked spinach is an incredibly nutrient-dense option and I recommend it frequently as a side dish. In traditional Chinese medicine, spinach is thought to have cooling properties and is used to reduce inflammation and tonify the blood.

AT A GLANCE: folate, iron, vitamin A

HEALING POWER: Spinach is well known for its high iron content, a nutrient that is rare among plant-based foods. Although spinach is high in iron, and calcium, these nutrients are not very well absorbed because of the high levels of oxalic acid in spinach. Oxalic acid binds to calcium and iron, making it harder for the body to absorb them. Spinach is full of antioxidant-rich vitamins A and C. These antioxidants fight free radicals and reduce inflammation. They also support the immune system by protecting against bacteria, toxins, and viruses. Dietary fiber helps promote optimal digestion and slows absorption of sugar into the bloodstream.

HEALTH BENEFITS/MEDICAL CONDITIONS: Spinach is great for bone health thanks to its high vitamin K content, as well as the absorbable portions of calcium and iron. The high beta-carotene and antioxidant levels in spinach protect against cancer and support the immune system. Spinach contains folate, which is especially beneficial for pregnant women because it helps prevent neural tube defects, such as spina bifida, in their babies. The dietary fiber in spinach may help promote normal blood sugar in those with diabetes and prediabetes.

CONSUMPTION: ½ cup cooked spinach, or 2 cups raw spinach

PEACHY HEMP GREEN SMOOTHIE

Serves 1

Prep time: 5 minutes

Green smoothies are my favorite breakfast option. If you don't love eating spinach, blending some into a smoothie may be an easy way for you to increase your intake. Adding spinach to a smoothie maintains all the veggie's benefits, without the bitter taste. It is important to ensure there is a balance of fruit, vegetables, healthy fat, and protein in your smoothies. In this recipe, chia seeds and hemp seeds add healthy fats and protein to keep you satisfied.

INGREDIENTS

¾ cup unsweetened plain almond milk, plus more as needed

½ banana, peeled and frozen

½ cup fresh baby spinach

¼ cup frozen peach slices

1 tablespoon chia seeds

1 tablespoon hemp seeds

1 teaspoon maple syrup

3 or 4 ice cubes

In a high-speed blender, combine the almond milk, banana, spinach, peaches, chia seeds, hemp seeds, maple syrup, and ice. Blend on high speed until smooth, adding more almond milk, if needed, to achieve your desired consistency.

INGREDIENT TIP

For smoothies, I recommend removing ripe bananas from their peel, cutting them in half, and freezing them in a freezer-safe container or bag. Using half a banana contributes adequate sweetness and creaminess without an overwhelming flavor or too much sugar.

VARIATION TIP

If you don't have hemp seeds, increase the chia seeds to 2 tablespoons.

Per Serving: Calories: 304; Saturated Fat: 1g; Total Fat: 16g; Protein: 11g; Total Carbs: 31g; Fiber: 10g; Sodium: 285mg

CLASSIC SAUTÉED GARLIC SPINACH

Serves 4 to 6
Prep time: 10 minutes
Cook time: 5 minutes

This versatile side dish can be enjoyed on its own or used as the base of a larger dish. Quick-cooking spinach (sautéing, stir-frying, or blanching) helps retain many of its water-soluble nutrients, as opposed to steaming or boiling them away.

INGREDIENTS

2 tablespoons extra-virgin olive oil

3 garlic cloves, finely minced

1½ pounds fresh baby spinach

Salt

Freshly ground black pepper

Lemon wedge (optional)

1. In a large pot over medium heat, heat the olive oil. Add the garlic and sauté for about 1 minute until fragrant.

2. Add the spinach and toss with the garlic and oil. Cook the spinach for 2 to 3 minutes, stirring constantly, until wilted. Season with salt and pepper.

3. Serve with a squeeze of lemon juice (if using).

INGREDIENT TIP

Choose leaves that are crisp and dark green. Avoid any leaves that are limp, damaged, contain yellow spots, or have a slimy coating.

Per Serving: Calories: 102; Saturated Fat: 1g; Total Fat: 8g; Protein: 5g; Total Carbs: 7g; Fiber: 4g; Sodium: 173mg

RADICCHIO

Commonly used in Italian cooking, radicchio is a bright white and red leafy vegetable known for its bitter, nutty taste. Radicchio is a form of chicory, which has been used medicinally for centuries. In South Africa, chicory syrup is used as a tonic for infants. In Turkey, chicory was historically used to make an ointment to promote wound healing. If you've ever purchased a "spring mix" in the salad aisle, you will identify radicchio as the sharp, bitter-tasting component. There are many varieties of radicchio, including the two varieties you will likely find at your local market: Treviso and Chioggia. The large, round, maroon-colored Chioggia varietal is the most widely available one in the United States.

AT A GLANCE: vitamins C, E, and K

HEALING POWER: Radicchio's purple color can be attributed to the flavonoid anthocyanin. Berries and other purple-colored plants like radicchio produce anthocyanins to protect themselves against stressors such as light, temperature fluctuations, and drought. The exact mechanism for how the compounds work in the human body is not clear, but they are shown to have antioxidant and anti-inflammatory effects. Anthocyanins may work in various ways to prevent cancer cell growth and proliferation.

HEALTH BENEFITS/MEDICAL CONDITIONS: Radicchio is a great vegetable for weight loss as it is high in fiber and low in calories. High vitamin K content may boost bone and heart health. Radicchio is rich in immune-boosting vitamin C, too. The anthocyanins in radicchio may protect against cancer, cardiovascular disease, and cognitive decline.

CONSUMPTION: 1 cup cooked

BALSAMIC ROASTED RADICCHIO

Serves 4

Prep time: 5 minutes

Cook time: 15 minutes

Roasting radicchio mellows its bitter, spicy flavor and the balsamic vinegar adds a hint of sweetness. This side dish is a fun way to mix up the flavors of your typical cooked leafy vegetables, such as spinach and kale. I recommend pairing the nutty, roasted radicchio with a hearty grain such as farro or brown rice.

INGREDIENTS

2 medium radicchio heads, quartered

¼ cup extra-virgin olive oil

Salt

Freshly ground black pepper

¼ cup balsamic vinegar

2 tablespoon chopped fresh basil

1. Preheat the oven to 400°F. Line a baking sheet with parchment paper.

2. Place the radicchio on the prepared baking sheet. Drizzle with the olive oil, toss to coat, and season with salt and pepper.

3. Roast for about 15 minutes, or until the radicchio leaves are slightly charred.

4. Transfer to a platter and drizzle with the vinegar and top with basil.

VARIATION TIP

You can use a regular balsamic vinegar for this recipe, or you can amp up the flavor with a more concentrated reduced balsamic. Bring 1 cup balsamic vinegar to a boil in a small pot, then reduce the heat and simmer it for 10 to 15 minutes.

Per Serving: Calories: 142; Saturated Fat: 2g; Total Fat: 13g; Protein: 2g; Total Carbs: 6g; Fiber: 2g; Sodium: 70mg

RADICCHIO, CANNELLINI BEAN, AND ENDIVE SALAD

Serves 4

Prep time: 5 minutes

Cook time: 15 minutes

This easy and flavorful warm salad is incredibly satisfying. Cannellini beans, also known as northern beans or white kidney beans, are a great plant-based source of protein with a meaty flavor. Cooked radicchio adds a smoky flavor to the dish without lots of sodium or calories.

INGREDIENTS

¼ cup extra-virgin olive oil

2 garlic cloves, finely minced

2 radicchio heads, chopped

1 endive head, chopped

1 (15-ounce) can no-salt-added cannellini beans, drained and rinsed

Salt

Freshly ground black pepper

1. In a large skillet over medium heat, heat the olive oil. Add the garlic and sauté for 1 minute until fragrant.

2. Add the radicchio and endive. Cook for about 5 minutes, stirring frequently, until softened.

3. Stir in the cannellini beans. Cook for 3 to 5 minutes, or until the cannellini beans are warmed. Season with salt and pepper. Serve warm.

INGREDIENT TIP

Choosing no-salt-added canned beans is a great way to cut cooking time. If you prefer to cook dried beans, soak the beans in water for at least 4 hours, or overnight, to break down some of the gas-causing complex sugars.

Per Serving: Calories: 230; Saturated Fat: 2g; Total Fat: 13g; Protein: 8g; Total Carbs: 23g; Fiber: 10g; Sodium: 82mg

KALE

Kale has been cultivated for more than 4,000 years and was used by the Romans as a treatment for digestive ailments. A cruciferous vegetable like broccoli, cabbage, and Brussels sprouts, kale comes in many varieties. It's a great food for various medical conditions, a well-balanced diet, and weight loss. You can increase your absorption of the fat-soluble vitamins—A, D, E, and K—in kale by massaging the kale in a salad with extra-virgin olive oil.

AT A GLANCE: beta-carotene, calcium, quercetin, vitamins C and K

HEALING POWER: Kale is packed with antioxidants such as beta-carotene, vitamin C, and flavonoids. Two flavonoids in particular, quercetin and kaempferol, are found in kale and help fight oxidative damage caused by free radicals in the body, reducing the risk of many diseases. Interestingly, kale contains a small amount of the omega-3 fatty acid called alpha-linolenic acid. This plant-based form of healthy fat is also found in walnuts and is considered neuroprotective and may reduce the risk of stroke. Research shows that kale's properties can also reduce cholesterol in the body. Kale and other cruciferous vegetables contain bile acid sequestrants, which work in the body to bind and eliminate bile acids through the digestive system. Bile acids are made from cholesterol, so an overall reduction in bile acids reduces cholesterol levels. Kale is a leafy green high in calcium. Unlike spinach, kale has low levels of oxalates, making the calcium more bioavailable.

HEALTH BENEFITS/MEDICAL CONDITIONS: The calcium in kale may help strengthen bones and it is good for children, pregnant women, and the elderly in this regard. Kale may be a good calcium source for those who are lactose intolerant. Lutein in kale may promote eye health and prevent cataracts. It may also protect the eyes from ultraviolet light damage. Kale contains various cancer-protective nutrients including fiber and antioxidants. The leafy green vegetable may lower cholesterol levels in the body, leading to a reduced risk of heart disease. Kale is a great high-fiber, low-calorie food that can promote weight loss and weight management.

CONSUMPTION: 2 cups raw, or 1 cup cooked

KALE WALNUT PESTO

Makes about 1 cup

Prep time: 10 minutes

Using kale and walnuts in place of traditional basil and pine nuts in pesto switches up the flavor and adds powerful nutrients. Walnuts look like brains and are good for your brain, as well, thanks to their high concentrations of DHA, an omega-3 fatty acid that has been shown to improve cognitive performance. Did you know that kale also contains omega-3s in the form of alpha-linolenic acid? Making this recipe is a no-brainer (pun intended)!

INGREDIENTS

½ bunch kale, stemmed and leaves chopped

½ cup roughly chopped raw unsalted walnuts

¼ cup extra-virgin olive oil, plus more
   as needed

¼ cup nutritional yeast

2 tablespoons freshly squeezed lemon juice

2 garlic cloves, peeled

Salt

Freshly ground black pepper

In a food processor or blender, combine the kale, walnuts, olive oil, nutritional yeast, lemon juice, and garlic. Blend until smooth, stopping to scrape down the sides with a spatula, as needed. Taste and season with salt and pepper. Add more olive oil, if needed, for a looser consistency.

INGREDIENT TIP

Choosing raw nuts preserves the healthy monounsaturated and polyunsaturated fats in them. Exposure to high heat can cause the fats to oxidize, which results in the formation of harmful free radicals and a rancid taste.

Per Serving (1 tablespoon): Calories: 77; Saturated Fat: 1g; Total Fat: 6g; Protein: 3g; Total Carbs: 4g; Fiber: 2g; Sodium: 21mg

"CHEESY" KALE CHIPS

Serves 4

Prep time: 10 minutes

Cook time: 30 minutes

Homemade kale chips are a crunchy, satisfying snack with tons of vitamins and minerals. Nutritional yeast adds a delicious "cheesy" flavor and provides vegan sources of protein and vitamin B_{12}. Many vegan and vegetarian diets are lacking in vitamin B_{12}, which is essential for DNA synthesis, red blood cell production, and nervous system health.

INGREDIENTS

1 bunch curly kale, stemmed and leaves roughly torn into pieces

2 tablespoons extra-virgin olive oil

¼ cup nutritional yeast

½ teaspoon garlic powder

Sea salt

1. Preheat the oven to 300°F. Line two rimmed baking sheets with parchment paper.

2. In a large bowl, massage the kale leaves with the olive oil.

3. Sprinkle the leaves with nutritional yeast, garlic powder, and a pinch salt. Massage the kale leaves again to distribute the seasonings. Place the leaves onto the prepared baking sheets, spacing them evenly in a single layer and not overcrowding.

4. Bake for 25 to 30 minutes, or until crispy. Let cool for 5 minutes.

STORAGE TIP

Store cooled kale chips in a container at room temperature for 2 to 3 days.

Per Serving: Calories: 187; Saturated Fat: 1g; Total Fat: 8g; Protein: 12g; Total Carbs: 21g; Fiber: 8g; Sodium: 75mg

BRUSSELS SPROUTS

Brussels sprouts are a member of the *Brassica* genus, which includes other cruciferous vegetables like kale and cauliflower. The veggie got its name from the city in which they were cultivated—Brussels, Belgium. This powerful vegetable resembles a mini cabbage and is well known for its cancer-fighting properties.

AT A GLANCE: glucosinolates, vitamins C and K

HEALING POWER: Brussels sprouts are rich in vitamin K, a vitamin necessary for bone and blood health. Vitamin K is a fat-soluble vitamin that helps blood clot properly. Brussels sprouts are also very high in dietary fiber. The fiber works as a scrub brush in the intestines, promoting optimal digestion. Dietary fiber also binds to cholesterol in the body and helps remove it. Vitamin C fights cancer-causing free radicals, neutralizing them and stopping their proliferation. Note that Brussels sprouts are known for their gas-producing properties. Brussels sprouts contain a group of sulfur-containing phytochemicals called glucosinolates, which may protect cells from DNA damage and protect against oxidative stress.

HEALTH BENEFITS/MEDICAL CONDITIONS: The high vitamin K content of Brussels sprouts makes them great for people with osteoporosis or any other bone-related disease, but people who take blood thinners such as warfarin need to watch their vitamin K intake to ensure they get the same amount every day. Brussels sprouts are great for digestive-related diseases, such as diverticulosis and constipation, but they may cause gas and bloating for those who have trouble breaking down the high fiber content. The high vitamin C level in Brussels sprouts may protect against cancer and boost the immune system. Glucosinolates may help prevent cancer and help reduce inflammation.

CONSUMPTION: 1 cup cooked or raw

CRISPY SPICY BRUSSELS SPROUTS

Serves 3

Prep time: 10 minutes

Cook time: 40 minutes

These spicy baked Brussels sprouts are prepared with avocado oil, a great high-heat alternative to typical vegetable oils because it has an extremely high smoke point, which helps avoid unnecessary toxins.

INGREDIENTS

3 cups trimmed, halved Brussels sprouts

3 tablespoons avocado oil, or extra-virgin olive oil

Salt

Freshly ground black pepper

3 tablespoons soy sauce, or coconut aminos

2 tablespoons maple syrup

1 tablespoon freshly squeezed lemon juice

1 garlic clove, minced

1 teaspoon sriracha

1. Preheat the oven to 400°F. Line a baking sheet with parchment paper or a silicone baking mat.

2. In a large bowl, stir together the Brussels sprouts and avocado oil. Season with salt and pepper. Spread the Brussels sprouts on the prepared baking sheet in a single layer.

3. Roast for 35 to 40 minutes, stirring or shaking the pan every 15 minutes to ensure even cooking.

4. While the Brussels sprouts roast, in a small skillet over medium-high heat, stir together the soy sauce, maple syrup, lemon juice, garlic, and sriracha. Cook for about 5 minutes, stirring constantly, until the sauce is thickened.

5. When the Brussels sprouts are cooked, transfer them to a bowl, pour in the sauce, and toss to coat.

VARIATION TIP

Coconut aminos is a great soy sauce substitute. If you are sensitive to gluten, be sure to use a gluten-free soy sauce.

Per Serving: Calories: 209; Saturated Fat: 2g; Total Fat: 14g; Protein: 4g; Total Carbs: 19g; Fiber: 4g; Sodium: 98mg

MAPLE MISO DIJON BRUSSELS SPROUTS

Serves 4

Prep time: 25 minutes
Cook time: 15 minutes

The savory, umami flavor of this dish is brought out by the miso, which is made from fermented soybeans. As a fermented food, miso is a great source of beneficial bacteria that promote optimal gut health.

INGREDIENTS

1 pound Brussels sprouts, trimmed and halved

5 tablespoons extra-virgin olive oil, divided

Salt

Freshly ground black pepper

2 tablespoons Dijon mustard

2 tablespoons sweet (white) miso

1 tablespoon maple syrup

1 tablespoon apple cider vinegar

1 tablespoon water

1. Preheat the oven to 425°F.

2. Place the Brussels sprouts on a large rimmed sheet pan and toss with 2 tablespoons of olive oil. Season with salt and pepper.

3. Roast for 15 minutes until the sprouts are tender and browned.

4. In a small bowl, whisk the remaining 3 tablespoons of olive oil, the mustard, miso, maple syrup, vinegar, and water until blended. Season with salt and pepper.

5. Drizzle half the maple miso dressing over the Brussels sprouts, adjusting the seasoning and adding more dressing, as needed.

STORAGE TIP

Refrigerate extra dressing in an airtight container for 3 to 4 days. Drizzle the dressing over salads and grains for a delicious treat!

Per Serving: Calories: 241; Saturated Fat: 3g; Total Fat: 19g; Protein: 5g; Total Carbs: 18g; Fiber: 5g; Sodium: 371mg

CAULIFLOWER

Along with broccoli and cabbage, cauliflower, another member of the *Brassica* genus, has been used for centuries to prevent cancer. Demand for cauliflower has risen over the past few years with various products coming to market, including cauliflower pizza crust, cauliflower rice, and even cauliflower chips. Using cauliflower as a substitute for high-fat foods and refined grains is a great way to promote weight loss and prevent common inflammatory diseases such as obesity, diabetes, and heart disease.

AT A GLANCE: choline, indoles, sulforaphane, vitamin C

HEALING POWER: Cauliflower contains powerful anti-inflammatory and antioxidant components, including vitamins C and K, and even some omega-3 fatty acids. It contains various glucosinolates, or enzymes, that stimulate the body's natural detoxification system. Two glucosinolates, sulforaphane and indole, are of particular interest. Sulforaphane is a sulfur-rich compound that acts as an antioxidant in the body, reducing inflammation and protecting cells against cancer-causing carcinogens. The phytonutrient indole prevents cells from growing and spreading, acting as an anticancer agent, specifically in hormone-dependent cancers. Cauliflower is also important for the brain. The essential nutrient choline plays a huge role in supporting metabolism, brain development, and cell health.

HEALTH BENEFITS/MEDICAL CONDITIONS: The glucosinolates in brassicas, including cauliflower, may help prevent cancer, especially breast, prostate, endometrial, and colon cancer. Although cauliflower can be hard for some people to digest, the high fiber and water content help promote a healthy digestive tract. Fiber and water also help prevent constipation. Increased fiber intake, such as that from cauliflower, is associated with a reduced risk of various diseases such as diabetes, obesity, and heart disease. The antioxidant power of cauliflower reduces cancer risk and decreases overall inflammation. Cauliflower is a great food for weight loss, as it is very low in carbohydrates and sugar, and incredibly filling thanks to the fiber it contains.

CONSUMPTION: 1 cup raw or cooked

CITRUS QUINOA AND CAULIFLOWER SALAD

Serves 2
Prep time: 20 minutes
Cook time: 30 minutes

Mix up your typical quinoa salad with citrus, chickpeas, and roasted cauliflower. Chickpeas and quinoa are rich in energy-boosting iron, which the vitamin C in the orange and cauliflower will help you absorb.

FOR THE SALAD

1 cup cauliflower florets

1 cup cooked chickpeas

2 tablespoons extra-virgin olive oil

¼ teaspoon ground cumin

2 cups cooked quinoa, cooled

1 navel orange, peeled, segmented, and each segment cut into thirds

2 tablespoons finely chopped red onion

FOR THE DRESSING

¼ cup extra-virgin olive oil

2 tablespoons apple cider vinegar

1 tablespoon Dijon mustard

1 teaspoon honey

INGREDIENT TIP

If you're not a fan of citrus or avoid acidic foods, swap the orange for ¼ cup unsweetened raisins.

TO MAKE THE SALAD

1. Preheat the oven to 375°F. Line a baking sheet with parchment paper and set aside.

2. In a large bowl, combine the cauliflower, chickpeas, olive oil, and cumin. Toss to coat. Transfer the cauliflower and chickpeas to the prepared baking sheet, spreading them into a single layer.

3. Roast for 30 minutes, or until the cauliflower and chickpeas are softened and golden brown. Let cool.

TO MAKE THE DRESSING

While the chickpeas and cauliflower roast, in a small bowl, whisk the olive oil, vinegar, mustard, and honey to blend. Set aside.

TO FINISH THE SALAD

Once cooled, in a large bowl, combine the cooked chickpeas and cauliflower, quinoa, orange segments, and red onion. Drizzle the dressing over the salad and toss to combine.

Per Serving: Calories: 796; Saturated Fat: 6g; Total Fat: 49g; Protein: 18g; Total Carbs: 79g; Fiber: 15g; Sodium: 124mg

BLUEBERRY CAULIFLOWER SMOOTHIE

Serves 1

Prep time: 5 minutes

Cauliflower is great substitute for bananas in smoothies, creating a creamy texture while reducing sugar and carbohydrate content. This smoothie will have you feeling full for hours and can help reduce your sugar cravings.

INGREDIENTS

1 cup unsweetened plain almond milk, plus more as needed

½ cup frozen cauliflower rice

½ cup frozen blueberries

2 tablespoons chia seeds

½ teaspoon vanilla extract

½ teaspoon ground cinnamon

3 or 4 ice cubes, plus more as needed

In a high-speed blender, combine the almond milk, cauliflower rice, blueberries, chia seeds, vanilla, cinnamon, and ice. Blend until smooth. Add more ice or almond milk, as needed, to create your desired consistency.

INGREDIENT TIP

If you can't tolerate raw cauliflower, try steaming and cooling the cauliflower rice before using it in the smoothie. Cooking makes the cauliflower easier to digest and can prevent uncomfortable gas. Not ready to fully embrace cauliflower in a smoothie? Substitute ½ banana for ¼ cup frozen cauliflower rice.

Per Serving: Calories: 216; Saturated Fat: 1g; Total Fat: 11g; Protein: 6g; Total Carbs: 23g; Fiber: 11g; Sodium: 378mg

BROCCOLI

In traditional Chinese medicine, broccoli is known for improving energy and clearing heat. Its "cooling" properties are used to promote eye health. Broccoli contains beta-carotene, which promotes eye, bone, and digestive health.

AT A GLANCE: calcium, folate, indole-3-carbinol, sulforaphane, vitamin C

HEALING POWER: Broccoli is full of glucosinolates, including indole-3-carbinol (I3C) and sulforaphane. These compounds work to interrupt the progression of cancer and prevent cancer in various ways. Studies show that I3C stops the progression of estrogen-enhanced tumors. Sulforaphane fights against cancer in another way, helping boost production of anticancer enzymes. Vitamin C and beta-carotene in broccoli also contribute their antioxidant effects to make broccoli an incredible cancer-fighting veggie. Broccoli is a great plant-based source of calcium. The primary role of calcium in the body is to support bone health, but it acts in many other ways, including helping the heart keep a normal rhythm and supporting the nerves that signal muscles to relax and contract. It should be noted that broccoli contains oxalates, which hinder the calcium from being readily absorbed by the body.

HEALTH BENEFITS/MEDICAL CONDITIONS: Broccoli contains multiple cancer-fighting compounds, including I3C, sulforaphane, and vitamin C. I3C may prevent the development of cancers related to estrogen, such as breast, endometrial, and cervical cancers. The vitamin C in broccoli may also boost immunity and be your best ally during cold and flu season. The calcium in broccoli is beneficial for people with osteoporosis and for pregnant women. Broccoli is a great source of nondairy calcium, especially for vegans or anyone who is lactose intolerant. Pregnant women may also benefit from the folate content in broccoli, which is essential for tissue growth and prevention of neural tube defects in babies. Broccoli is a great source of fiber and may help protect against constipation, high cholesterol, obesity, and heart disease.

CONSUMPTION: 1 cup cooked or raw

BROCCOLI AND ARUGULA SOUP

Serves 4
Prep time: 20 minutes
Cook time: 20 minutes

Soup doesn't get much simpler than this peppery broccoli and arugula mix. Puréeing vegetables can help you eat more of them, as the blending process essentially pre-digests and breaks down the fiber, which makes them easier on your digestive system. Vitamin C is typically leached out of broccoli during boiling. By blending the cooking liquid into the soup, you preserve broccoli's naturally high vitamin C content.

INGREDIENTS

2 tablespoons extra-virgin olive oil

½ yellow onion, chopped

1 garlic clove, finely minced

2 cups fresh or frozen broccoli florets

2 cups low-sodium vegetable broth

1 cup arugula

Salt

Freshly ground black pepper

1. In a medium saucepan over medium heat, heat the olive oil. Add the onion and garlic and sauté for 1 minute until fragrant. Add the broccoli and sauté for 4 to 5 minutes, or until bright green.

2. Add the vegetable broth and bring the mixture to a boil. Reduce the heat to maintain a simmer and cook for 5 to 8 minutes, or until the broccoli is tender. Let cool for 5 minutes, as you need to be careful when blending hot liquids.

3. Carefully transfer the soup to a high-speed blender. Add the arugula and blend until smooth. Taste and season with salt and pepper.

VARIATION TIP

Want a more complete meal? Add some protein and healthy fats by sprinkling 2 tablespoons chopped nuts and seeds on your soup. I recommend pumpkin seeds or pine nuts.

Per Serving: Calories: 91; Saturated Fat: 1g; Total Fat: 7g; Protein: 3g; Total Carbs: 5g; Fiber: 2g; Sodium: 91mg

STIR-FRY BROCCOLI "RICE"

Serves 2
Prep time: 15 minutes
Cook time: 5 minutes

Broccoli "rice" is a great low-carb, high-fiber alternative to traditional white rice and adds extra nutrients like calcium to your meal. Note that the broccoli stalk and stems are included in this recipe. The broccoli stem is highly nutritious and contains even more calcium, iron, and vitamin C than the florets do.

INGREDIENTS

1 broccoli head, cut into florets, stem peeled and cut into chunks

2 tablespoons avocado oil

1 tablespoon minced peeled fresh ginger

1 garlic clove, finely minced

1 cup frozen shelled edamame

1 large carrot, finely chopped

2 tablespoons water

1 tablespoon low-sodium soy sauce, or coconut aminos

INGREDIENT TIP

If you're short on time, use frozen broccoli. Many supermarkets now carry frozen and fresh "riced" broccoli and cauliflower. These are great options to keep in the freezer for a quick and easy dish!

1. In a food processor, process the broccoli florets and stems until they resemble a rice consistency.

2. In a large skillet over medium heat, heat the avocado oil. Add the ginger and garlic and cook for about 1 minute until fragrant.

3. Add the broccoli "rice," edamame, carrot, and water. Stir to mix and cover the skillet with a lid. Steam for 3 to 4 minutes, or until the broccoli is well cooked.

4. Stir in the soy sauce and serve hot.

SUBSTITUTION TIP

If you're not a fan of broccoli, use cauliflower in this recipe. Be sure to add the cauliflower stems (if using fresh cauliflower). To prepare, use a vegetable peeler to peel away the outer layer of the stem, then slice the remaining stem flesh into chunks before "ricing" in the food processor.

Per Serving: Calories: 298; Saturated Fat: 2g; Total Fat: 18g; Protein: 14g; Total Carbs: 28g; Fiber: 10g; Sodium: 451mg

ACORN SQUASH

Acorn squash is a deliciously sweet source of complex carbohydrates. It's part of the winter squash family called cucurbitaceae that includes butternut squash and pumpkin. Squashes are generally divided into two categories, summer and winter, based on their harvest time.

AT A GLANCE: alpha-carotene, vitamins B_6 and C

HEALING POWER: You can tell by the orange color of the acorn squash flesh that it is a great source of carotenoids. Acorn squash is one of the best sources of alpha-carotene, a carotenoid shown to have high anticancer activity. Vitamin C is a water-soluble vitamin that fights infection and has strong antioxidant capabilities. It works against free radicals and toxins, helping eliminate them from the body to reduce the overall toxic load. Vitamin B_6, or pyridoxine, is needed in the body to maintain nerve, skin, and red blood cell health. It's a critical component for the nervous and immune systems.

HEALTH BENEFITS/MEDICAL CONDITIONS: Thanks to its high vitamin C and carotenoid content, acorn squash is beneficial for protecting against cancer. The fiber content in acorn squash may help protect against digestive issues such as constipation, irritable bowel syndrome, and colorectal cancer. Acorn squash is a great complex carbohydrate alternative to potatoes for those with diabetes, as it is high in fiber and has many vitamins and minerals. Acorn squash may be helpful for pregnant women suffering from morning sickness, as B_6 and carbohydrates have been shown to reduce the severity of nausea.

CONSUMPTION: 1 cup cooked acorn squash, about ½ acorn squash

CHICKPEA-STUFFED ACORN SQUASH

Serves 2

Prep time: 20 minutes

Cook time: 45 minutes

This easy fall meal comes together in minutes and the squash can be roasted ahead of time for a quick weeknight meal. Baking the squash retains the vitamin C, which offers a great boost to your immunity. Adding nutritional yeast lends a "cheesy" flavor and tons of B vitamins. Nutritional yeast is a fantastic plant-based source of B_{12}, which is critical for energy, DNA production, and an overall healthy nervous system!

INGREDIENTS

2 tablespoons extra-virgin olive oil, divided

1 acorn squash, halved and seeded

1 teaspoon garlic powder

Salt

Freshly ground black pepper

2 garlic cloves, finely minced

1 tomato, cut into ¼-inch dice

1 globe eggplant, cut into ¼-inch dice

1 (15-ounce) can no-salt-added chickpeas, drained and rinsed

1 cup low-sugar tomato sauce

2 to 4 tablespoons nutritional yeast

Red pepper flakes, for seasoning (optional)

1. Preheat the oven to 400°F. Line a baking sheet with parchment paper.

2. Using 1 tablespoon of olive oil, rub some into each squash half. Sprinkle each half with garlic powder, salt, and pepper. Place the squash, flesh-side down, on the prepared baking sheet.

3. Bake for 45 minutes, flipping the squash flesh-side up halfway through the baking time.

4. While the squash bakes, in a medium sauté pan or skillet over medium heat, heat the remaining 1 tablespoon of olive oil. Add the garlic and cook for about 20 seconds until fragrant.

5. Add the tomato and eggplant (and 1 to 2 tablespoons of water, if the vegetables stick to pan) and cook for 3 to 5 minutes, or until soft.

6. Stir in the chickpeas and tomato sauce. Reduce the heat to low and cook for about 2 minutes, or until the chickpeas and tomato sauce are warm.

INGREDIENT TIP

Don't throw out the squash seeds! Acorn squash seeds (and other squash varieties) are packed with protein, heart-healthy fats, and fiber! Roast them with olive oil and a dash salt for a quick nutritious snack or salad topper.

7. Stuff each squash half with 1 cup of the chickpea ragout. Top with 1 to 2 tablespoons of nutritional yeast and sprinkle with red pepper flakes (if using).

Per Serving: Calories: 570; Saturated Fat: 2g; Total Fat: 19g; Protein: 25g; Total Carbs: 87g; Fiber: 28g; Sodium: 111mg

ACORN SQUASH AND SWEET POTATO MASH

Serves 3 or 4

Prep time: 15 minutes

Cook time: 40 minutes

This mash makes a great substitute for regular mashed potatoes. The acorn squash and sweet potato amp up the nutrition, providing more vitamin A and C than white potatoes. Coconut oil is a good source of the medium-chain fatty acid lauric acid, which, research suggests, may protect against Alzheimer's disease.

INGREDIENTS

1 acorn squash, halved, seeded, and cut into
  ½-inch-thick half-moons

1 medium sweet potato, peeled and cut into
  ½-inch cubes

2 tablespoons coconut oil, melted

Salt

Freshly ground black pepper

¼ cup unsweetened plain almond milk

2 tablespoons chopped fresh chives

SUBSTITUTION TIP

If acorn squash is not in season or isn't available where you live, you can make this mash with 2 sweet potatoes, or substitute butternut squash for the acorn squash.

1. Preheat the oven to 350°F. Line a baking sheet with parchment paper and set aside.

2. In a large bowl, toss together the squash, sweet potato, and melted coconut oil to coat. Season with salt and pepper. Transfer the vegetables to the prepared baking sheet and spread them into a single layer.

3. Bake for 30 to 40 minutes, or until the vegetables are soft and lightly brown. Transfer the cooked sweet potato to a large bowl.

4. Using a large spoon, separate the cooked acorn squash flesh from the skin. Discard the skin and add the flesh to bowl with the sweet potato.

5. Add the almond milk. Using a potato masher, mash the potato and squash until well combined. Taste and season with salt and pepper. Serve hot, garnished with chives.

Per Serving: Calories: 178; Saturated Fat: 8g; Total Fat: 9g; Protein: 2g; Total Carbs: 23g; Fiber: 4g; Sodium: 98mg

PUMPKINS

In traditional Chinese medicine, pumpkin is used to treat eczema, edema, and diabetes. Cooked pumpkin and its seeds are used as an antiparasitic. Pumpkin seeds are rich in healthy fats, fiber, protein, and antioxidants. Pop them into the oven with some olive oil and salt for a healthy, healing snack.

AT A GLANCE: beta-carotene, potassium, vitamin C

HEALING POWER: Pumpkins are incredibly high in beta-carotene, the carotenoid that your body actively converts into vitamin A. This carotenoid works as an antioxidant, protecting your cells against damage and oxidizing free radicals. Vitamin A, along with vitamin C, helps strengthen the immune system. Pumpkin is also great for the skin because of its vitamin A and C content. Carotenoids can help protect the skin cells against sun damage, as they may absorb ultraviolet light. The body also uses vitamin C to create collagen, which can decrease as you age.

HEALTH BENEFITS/MEDICAL CONDITIONS: Vitamins A and C in pumpkin are great immune system boosters. Pumpkin is great for those seeking weight management because it is low in calories and high in fiber. Pumpkin may be cancer-protective thanks to its high antioxidant levels, especially carotenoids. The vitamins in pumpkin, particularly vitamins A, C, and E, promote optimal skin health. Vitamin C–rich pumpkin can work in tandem with protein to create more collagen, which benefits those with osteoarthritis and joint pain.

CONSUMPTION: 1 cup cooked

PUMPKIN PIE GREEN SMOOTHIE

Serves 1

Prep time: 5 minutes

This smoothie is pumpkin pie in a cup! The most important ingredients, aside from the vitamin A–rich pumpkin, are the chia seeds. Chia seeds are chock-full of protein and heart-healthy omega-3s. They expand in water, forming a gel that keeps you full and acts like a scrub brush in the gut.

INGREDIENTS

1 cup unsweetened plain almond milk

½ banana, peeled and frozen

½ cup pure pumpkin purée

½ cup frozen kale

1 tablespoon chia seeds

1 teaspoon pumpkin pie spice (or a mix of ginger, nutmeg, cloves, and/or allspice)

1 teaspoon maple syrup (optional)

½ teaspoon ground cinnamon

In a blender, combine the almond milk, banana, pumpkin, kale, chia seeds, pumpkin pie spice, maple syrup (if using), and cinnamon. Blend on high speed until smooth.

INGREDIENT TIP

I recommend purchasing canned pumpkin, which is just cooked, puréed pumpkin. It takes away a lot of the work of cutting and roasting a whole pumpkin. Note that the canned pumpkin is sometimes confused with pumpkin pie filling, which is sweetened and flavored with spices. Look for pure pumpkin.

Per Serving: Calories: 272; Saturated Fat: 1g; Total Fat: 11g; Protein: 8g; Total Carbs: 37g; Fiber: 14g; Sodium: 385mg

CHOCOLATE CHIP PUMPKIN BANANA BREAD

Serves 9
Prep time: 10 minutes
Cook time: 35 minutes

The smell of this delicious blender bread makes your mouth water! Perfect for a snack or dessert, this bread is loaded with fiber and may help those struggling with digestive issues or irritable bowel syndrome. Slather an extra bit of almond butter on top for a delicious, nutritious breakfast!

INGREDIENTS

Coconut oil, for preparing the baking pan

2 cups old-fashioned rolled oats

1½ bananas, peeled

½ cup pure pumpkin purée

¼ cup maple syrup

¼ cup almond butter (optional)

¼ cup unsweetened plain almond milk, or unsweetened vanilla almond milk

1 teaspoon baking soda

1 teaspoon baking powder

1 teaspoon ground cinnamon

½ teaspoon ground ginger

½ teaspoon ground nutmeg

¼ cup dark chocolate chips (at least 70 percent cacao)

1. Preheat the oven to 350°F. Coat a 9-by-5-inch loaf pan with coconut oil and set aside.

2. In a high-speed blender or food processor, combine the oats, bananas, pumpkin, maple syrup, almond butter (if using), almond milk, baking soda, baking powder, cinnamon, ginger, and nutmeg. Blend until well combined.

3. Pour the batter into the loaf pan, then mix in the chocolate chips.

4. Bake for 35 minutes, or until a knife inserted into the center comes out clean. Let cool and cut into 1-inch slices.

INGREDIENT TIP

Peel and freeze the remaining half of the banana to use for smoothies later on.

SUBSTITUTION TIP

If you don't have almond butter, use any other nut or seed butter, or leave it out.

Per Serving: Calories: 146; Saturated Fat: 1g; Total Fat: 3g; Protein: 3g; Total Carbs: 28g; Fiber: 3g; Sodium: 142mg

TOMATOES

Referred to as *pommes d'amour* or "love apples" by the French, tomatoes were once believed to have aphrodisiac power. They have a turbulent history in the United States, as many people thought tomatoes were toxic and caused "brain fever," appendicitis, and cancer. Little did people know that tomatoes are an incredible cancer fighter, providing ample amounts of vitamin C and lycopene. Cooked tomatoes may offer even more nutritional benefits than raw, but try to limit processed tomato products such as ketchup, tomato sauce, and tomato paste. Botanically speaking, a tomato is a fruit; however, it has been deemed a vegetable by law.

AT A GLANCE: lycopene, potassium, vitamins A and C

HEALING POWER: The red pigment of tomatoes comes from the powerful antioxidant lycopene. This antioxidant works to slow and stop the growth of cancer cells by neutralizing cell-damaging free radicals. Your cancer protection may increase if you cook your tomatoes, as lycopene levels have been shown to increase through cooking. The body's absorption of lycopene is also increased when combined with healthy fat sources, such as olive oil. According to the USDA, 1 cup of sliced tomatoes provides almost one-fourth of your daily vitamin C needs.

HEALTH BENEFITS/MEDICAL CONDITIONS: Because of their high amounts of lycopene and vitamin C, tomatoes may help prevent cancer. Lycopene is also great for skin care and is found in many over-the-counter products to soothe inflammation and protect against acne. Tomatoes are full of water, which hydrates inside and out. The vitamin C in tomatoes may help prevent colds. The calcium and vitamin K content help promote bone health. The potassium in tomatoes may benefit heart health and help reduce blood pressure. The vitamin A promotes skin, hair, nail, and eye health.

CONSUMPTION: 1 cup cooked or raw

QUICK RATATOUILLE

Serves 4
Prep time: 15 minutes
Cook time: 30 minutes

Did you know that cooking tomatoes increases the amount of the phytochemical lycopene that the vegetable has? Lycopene absorption is enhanced in the body by combining it with healthy fat sources such as olive oil. As a result, this ratatouille is a great way to reap all the benefits of tomatoes and the antioxidant lycopene in a deliciously simple dish.

INGREDIENTS

2 tablespoons extra-virgin olive oil

½ large yellow onion, chopped

2 garlic cloves, finely minced

1 eggplant, cut into ½-inch chunks

1 zucchini, cut into ½-inch chunks

1 yellow bell pepper, cut into ½-inch chunks

2 tomatoes, chopped

½ teaspoon dried rosemary

Salt

Freshly ground black pepper

1. In a large sauté pan or skillet over medium heat, heat the olive oil. Add the onion and garlic and cook for about 2 minutes, or until slightly browned.

2. Add the eggplant, zucchini, yellow bell pepper, tomatoes, and rosemary. Season with salt and pepper. Stir well and let simmer, uncovered, for 20 to 25 minutes, stirring again halfway through the cooking, until the vegetables are softened.

INGREDIENT TIP

A deep red color is a sign that the tomato has greater amounts of lycopene. Do not store tomatoes in the refrigerator, as they are sensitive to cold. If you need to speed the ripening process, store the tomatoes in a paper bag.

Per Serving: Calories: 127; Saturated Fat: 1g; Total Fat: 8g; Protein: 3g; Total Carbs: 15g; Fiber: 6g; Sodium: 51mg

MARINATED TOMATO ONION SALAD

Serves 3

Prep time: 10 minutes, plus 2 hours to marinate (optional)

There's nothing better than a late-summer tomato salad. Tomatoes and onions work synergistically. Research suggests the sulfur compounds in onions may boost the absorption of the antioxidant lycopene found in tomatoes.

INGREDIENTS

2 large tomatoes, cut into slices

1 sweet onion, thinly sliced

¼ cup extra-virgin olive oil

2 tablespoons red wine vinegar

1 teaspoon salt

½ teaspoon honey

¼ teaspoon garlic powder

Freshly ground black pepper

1. On a platter, arrange the sliced tomatoes and onions.

2. In a small bowl, whisk the olive oil, vinegar, salt, honey, and garlic powder to combine. Season with pepper and whisk again. Pour the dressing over the tomatoes and onions. Cover and let marinate in the refrigerator for at least 2 hours.

COOKING TIP

If you're short on time, no need to marinate the salad. You can serve it right away! I recommend pairing it with a nutty grain, such as farro or wheat berries.

Per Serving: Calories: 187; Saturated Fat: 2g; Total Fat: 17g; Protein: 2g; Total Carbs: 9g; Fiber: 2g; Sodium: 765mg

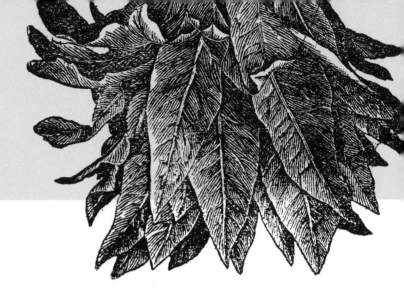

ALL HAIL THE KALE

Does it seem like everyone you know is crazy about kale? From kale crackers to kale-infused cocktails, the cruciferous vegetable is everywhere. Kale has gained popularity in recent years, but it has a long history. The leafy vegetable was popular in Roman and Greek times, when the ancient Greeks reportedly used the boiled leaves as a cure for drunkenness. The kale plant is incredibly versatile—Russians even produced a variety that could survive the brutal Russian winters. Kale arrived on the scene in the United States in the 1600s, but hit its heyday in the past decade. It has since been given a whole day of a celebration: The first Wednesday in October is National Kale Day! Celebrate the highly nutritious (and trendy) veggie by making some "Cheesy" Kale Chips (page 45)!

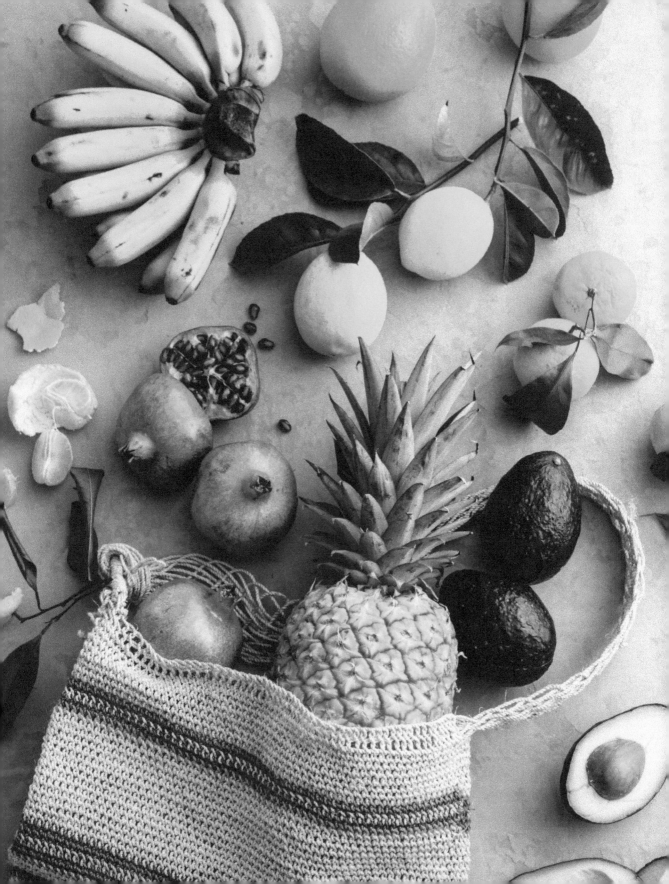

4

Fruits

Dubbed "nature's candy," fruit is a sweet and delicious way to enjoy the healing properties of plant-based foods. Fruits contain antioxidants, vitamins, and minerals that can help improve digestion, boost immunity, and give you a healthy glow. Throughout this section, we will look at profiles of 10 incredibly nutritious fruits, including citrus, berries, and avocado. The recipes highlight the versatility of each fruit and offer fun, inventive ways to use fruit in both sweet and savory dishes.

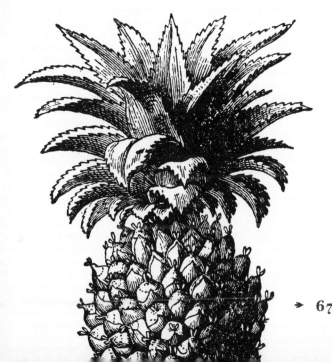

GRAPEFRUITS

Grapefruit is well known as a tangy, vitamin C–rich addition to breakfast, but grapefruit has many healing powers beyond the breakfast table. Many varieties of grapefruit are available, including the Ruby Red, which is popular for its bright color and sweet taste. Known for promoting weight loss, grapefruit has long been used by those looking to shed a few pounds. Grapefruit is also used as an ingredient in topical creams to reduce cellulite.

AT A GLANCE: folic acid, naringin, vitamin C

HEALING POWER: Grapefruit is high in fiber, low in calories, and full of hydrating water that can help fill you up. Grapefruit also contains compounds such as nootkatone, which contributes to the delicious citrus smell and appears to activate energy metabolism, promoting weight loss. Like other citrus fruits, grapefruit is high in vitamin C, which fights oxidation in the body and helps prevent the development of cancer cells. The flavonoid naringin found in the inner peel of grapefruit, has been shown to fight cancer by inhibiting tumor growth.

HEALTH BENEFITS/MEDICAL CONDITIONS: Consuming grapefruit is a great way to prevent obesity, promote weight loss, and boost metabolism. The fruit has a high fluid content that can help increase hydration and benefit skin health. Vitamin C plays a large role in collagen formation and can promote clear skin, boost immunity, and fight cancer. Folic acid, or folate, is important for women looking to conceive, or those who are pregnant, to prevent neural tube defects in the infant.

CONSUMPTION: 1 medium grapefruit

GRAPEFRUIT LIME ICE POPS

Makes 4 to 6 ice pops

Prep time: 5 minute, plus 4 hours freeze time

Making your own ice pops is a great (and sweet) way to meet your hydration needs and consume nutritious grapefruit. Blending grapefruit instead of juicing it preserves the fiber. Consuming fiber with the naturally sugary juice helps modulate the blood sugar response.

INGREDIENTS

2 Ruby Red grapefruits, or pink grapefruit, peeled, seeded, and pith removed

1 cup water

¼ cup honey (optional)

Juice of 1 lime

In a blender, combine the grapefruit, water, honey (if using), and lime juice. Blend on high speed for 1 minute, or until well combined. Pour the liquid into ice pop molds and freeze for at least 4 hours.

INGREDIENT TIP

Juice loses sweetness when frozen. These pops may not be very sweet, so you may need to increase the amount of honey as desired.

COOKING TIP

If you don't have ice pop molds, use small paper cups and ice pop sticks.

Per Serving: Calories: 29; Saturated Fat: 0g; Total Fat: 0g; Protein: 1g; Total Carbs: 8g; Fiber: 1g; Sodium: 0mg

GRAPEFRUIT AVOCADO SALAD

Serves 4

Prep time: 30 minutes

Anything tastes better with avocado—including grapefruit. This refreshing blend is an immune-boosting powerhouse! Both fruits are rich in vitamin C and the healthy fat content of avocados and olive oil helps promote absorption of the vitamin. Grapefruit zest adds a zing, but also fiber and phytochemicals.

INGREDIENTS

2 medium grapefruits

2 medium avocados, peeled, halved, pitted, and cut into slices

2 tablespoons extra-virgin olive oil

1 shallot, minced

1 teaspoon grated grapefruit zest

1 teaspoon white wine vinegar

Salt

Freshly ground black pepper

1. Using a sharp knife, cut the skin and white pith off the grapefruit. Holding the grapefruit over a bowl, cut between the membranes to release the grapefruit sections, reserving the juice.

2. On a plate, arrange the grapefruit sections and avocado slices, layering and alternating the fruits.

3. In a small bowl, whisk together 2 tablespoons of the reserved grapefruit juice, the olive oil, shallot, grapefruit zest, and vinegar. Drizzle the dressing onto the grapefruit and avocado. Season with salt and pepper.

COOKING TIP

Purchase already-sectioned grapefruit slices to save time on prep. Avocados turn brown quickly, so serve the salad within an hour or two of making it.

Per Serving: Calories: 247; Saturated Fat: 3g; Total Fat: 21g; Protein: 3g; Total Carbs: 18g; Fiber: 7g; Sodium: 46mg

ORANGES

Juicy, sweet oranges are known for their vitamin C, a nutrient widely used to fight the common cold. One medium orange can provide almost all the recommended vitamin C intake for the day. The orange peel has been used to make aromatherapy oil, which is used to help people with anxiety. In traditional Chinese medicine, oranges are used to promote digestion and improve appetite. From a nutrition standpoint, I recommend eating the whole orange as opposed to pouring a glass of orange juice, as the whole fruit contains all the beneficial fiber.

AT A GLANCE: fiber, limonene, vitamin C

HEALING POWER: The vitamin C in oranges helps support various pathogen-fighting cells in the body. It stimulates the production and function of white blood cells and helps the body produce antibodies that neutralize or eliminate viruses and bacteria. The skin is the first level of defense in the body, so it makes sense that vitamin C helps promote wound healing and build collagen. Vitamin C works as an antioxidant, blocking damage caused by free radicals. Limonene, another antioxidant found in oranges, may fight cancer by reducing the growth of tumors. According to the USDA, one large orange contains 4.4 grams of dietary fiber. This dietary fiber works to help eliminate cholesterol in the body and improve sluggish digestion.

HEALTH BENEFITS/MEDICAL CONDITIONS: Vitamin C in oranges can help improve immune system function and may help reduce the duration of cold symptoms. Vitamin C may also protect against heart disease and stroke and be beneficial for those struggling with osteoarthritis. Oranges can help prevent cancer thanks to their high amounts of vitamin C and other compounds such as limonene. The dietary fiber in oranges can improve digestive health and eliminate constipation. Fiber may also lower cholesterol, which can be beneficial for those at risk of heart disease. Oranges are a good fruit for weight loss, as they are hydrating and full of fiber, helping you feel fuller longer. Vitamin C has been shown to increase iron absorption, so in combination with iron-containing foods, oranges may be helpful in treating anemia.

CONSUMPTION: 1 medium orange

ZESTY SESAME-ORANGE VINAIGRETTE

Makes 1 cup

Prep time: 10 minutes

Sesame seeds are a great source of nondairy calcium and are the perfect complement to this Asian-inspired vinaigrette. Using the zest of the orange adds flavor, but also contributes a large amount of pectin, a soluble fruit fiber that can help relieve constipation, promote weight loss, and even offer anticancer benefits.

INGREDIENTS

Grated zest of 1 orange

Juice of 1 orange

2 tablespoons low-sodium soy sauce

2 tablespoons rice wine vinegar

2 tablespoons grated peeled fresh ginger

2 scallions, white parts only, minced

2 garlic cloves, minced

1 tablespoon honey

¼ cup avocado oil

2 tablespoons toasted sesame oil

Salt

Freshly ground black pepper

2 tablespoons sesame seeds, toasted (optional)

1. In a medium bowl, whisk the orange zest, orange juice, soy sauce, vinegar, ginger, scallions, garlic, and honey.

2. Slowly whisk in the avocado oil and sesame oil until blended. Taste and season with salt and pepper.

3. Whisk in the sesame seeds (if using) before serving.

INGREDIENT TIP

Sesame oil can be very expensive, but you can make it at home! In a skillet over medium heat, whisk ¼ cup of sesame seeds and 1 cup of a neutral oil, such as canola or safflower. Cook, stirring, until the seeds turn brown. Remove from the heat. Cool the oil, then blend until well combined. Let the oil rest for 2 hours before straining out the seed parts through a fine-mesh sieve set over a bowl.

Per Serving (2 tablespoons): Calories: 115; Saturated Fat: 1g; Total Fat: 10g; Protein: 1g; Total Carbs: 6g; Fiber: 1g; Sodium: 240mg

SPINACH SALAD WITH ORANGE SLICES AND TOASTED ALMONDS

Serves 2

Prep time: 10 minutes

Looking for ways to boost your iron levels? Vitamin C helps increase absorption of non-heme (plant-based) iron found in foods such as spinach and almonds. By adding orange to the salad, you boost both energy and focus.

INGREDIENTS

3 cups fresh baby spinach

1 orange, peeled and sectioned

½ cup chopped almonds

¼ cup Zesty Sesame-Orange Vinaigrette (page 72)

1. Place the spinach on a platter. Arrange the oranges on top of the spinach. Sprinkle the almonds over the salad.

2. Spoon the vinaigrette over the salad and serve.

INGREDIENT TIP

To avoid spoilage, do not wash the spinach before storing it. Smaller oranges are generally juicier than larger ones. Choose navel oranges with small navels, as the larger navels indicate the orange was overripe when picked.

Per Serving: Calories: 386; Saturated Fat: 3g; Total Fat: 29g; Protein: 11g; Total Carbs: 27g; Fiber: 9g; Sodium: 276mg

LEMONS

In the 1700s, lemons and limes were given to sailors at sea to prevent scurvy, a disease caused by vitamin C deficiency. Lemons appear frequently throughout history as a home remedy for indigestion, as lemon water is thought to neutralize stomach acid. Applied topically, lemon juice has been used to soothe sunburn and stop nosebleeds. The saying goes, "When life gives you lemons, make lemonade!" I would modify that and say make some hot water with lemon. You'll reap numerous benefits (with no sugar)!

AT A GLANCE: limonene, vitamin C

HEALING POWER: Lemons are known as natural detoxifiers and cold tonics. Like other citrus fruits, lemons contain high amounts of vitamin C, which helps white blood cells fight infection, thereby boosting immunity. Lemons are very helpful with wound healing, as vitamin C helps protect against harmful bacteria. Like oranges, lemons contain limonene, a component found in the peel that helps prevent cancer growth. Lemon water is a simple way to detoxify the body naturally, improving digestion and preventing the buildup of toxins.

HEALTH BENEFITS/MEDICAL CONDITIONS: The vitamin C content in lemons boosts the immune system, promotes wound healing, and fights cancer. Lemons may also protect against heart disease and stroke because of their high vitamin C content. Research suggests that consuming lemon on a daily basis, in combination with walking, can lower blood pressure. The sour taste of lemons, and even the fragrant smell, may help relieve pregnancy-related nausea. The fiber found in lemons, especially pectin, can help improve digestive issues.

CONSUMPTION: the juice of ½ lemon

LEMON GINGER COLD TONIC

Serves 1

Prep time: 5 minutes

Cook time: 10 minutes

The minute I feel a cold coming on, I brew this warming lemon ginger tonic. The combination of lemon, ginger, and honey has been used throughout history to treat cold and flu symptoms and soothe sore throats. Today, you can find lemon ginger shots in many juice shops and grocery stores, but this tonic is simple to make at home and you'll feel relief instantly.

INGREDIENTS

2 cups water

1 (½-inch) piece fresh ginger, peeled and grated

½ lemon

1 teaspoon honey

1. In a small pot, bring the water to a boil over high heat.

2. Add the ginger to the water and turn off the heat. Steep for 10 minutes.

3. Use a fine-mesh sieve set over a bowl to remove the ginger pieces from the water. Discard the ginger.

4. Squeeze the lemon juice into the ginger water and stir in the honey until dissolved.

VARIATION TIP

If you want to spice things up, add ⅛ teaspoon cayenne pepper. Cayenne is a natural decongestant, but beware: It can be very spicy—a little bit goes a long way!

Per Serving: Calories: 27; Saturated Fat: 0g; Total Fat: 0g; Protein: 0g; Total Carbs: 6g; Fiber: 0g; Sodium: 5mg

CLASSIC LEMON APPLE CIDER VINAIGRETTE

Makes 1 cup

Prep time: 5 minutes

This dressing is a staple in my house. I make a batch each week to use with salads and grains, and even as a marinade. With the lemon, raw honey, onion, and apple cider vinegar, this dressing adds a tasty detoxifying boost to any dish.

INGREDIENTS

⅓ cup extra-virgin olive oil

¼ cup raw apple cider vinegar

2 tablespoons freshly squeezed lemon juice

2 tablespoons raw honey

2 tablespoons Dijon mustard

1 tablespoon minced shallot

Salt

Freshly ground black pepper

In a glass jar with a lid, combine the olive oil, vinegar, lemon juice, honey, mustard, and shallot. Seal the lid and shake the jar until the ingredients are well combined. Taste and season with salt and pepper.

STORAGE TIP

Refrigerate, tightly sealed, for up to 1 week.

VARIATION TIP

If you don't have honey, use maple syrup in its place.

INGREDIENT TIP

Before cutting lemons, roll them back and forth on the counter while applying pressure with your hand. This helps break down the lemon and extracts more juice.

Per Serving (2 tablespoons): Calories: 94; Saturated Fat: 1g; Total Fat: 9g; Protein: 0g; Total Carbs: 5g; Fiber: 0g; Sodium: 65mg

APPLES

As the saying goes, "An apple a day keeps the doctor away." This may be incredibly true. Apples are known as prevention for tooth decay, as crunching on the fruit can help cleanse the mouth. Apples have been made into tonics like cider and vinegar for many years and are widely used in folk medicine to promote optimal digestion. Next time you reach for an apple, be sure to keep the skin intact, as the peel contains most of the fruit's fiber and antioxidants.

AT A GLANCE: pectin, quercetin, soluble fiber, vitamin C

HEALING POWER: Apples are a great source of fiber, including both soluble and insoluble fiber and pectin. The soluble and insoluble fiber can help you feel full, but they also expand in the digestive tract, helping move things along. Pectin forms a gel in the intestines, slowing digestion. Soluble fiber also acts like pectin, creating a gel-like consistency in the intestines, also helping lower cholesterol. The antioxidant quercetin is found abundantly in apples and works to protect cells from oxidation. This phenolic compound prevents inflammation and fights cancer. Vitamin C also provides important antioxidant protection for immune health (let's keep that doctor away)!

HEALTH BENEFITS/MEDICAL CONDITIONS: The high fiber content of apples can help decrease the risk of various chronic diseases, improve digestive health, and alleviate constipation. Insoluble fiber in apples helps prevent diverticulosis and relieve constipation. The antioxidant capacity of apples may lower the risk of heart disease and lung cancer. Evidence suggests the phytochemicals in apples may help protect against asthma. Apples are a great fiber-filled food to include in your diet to help manage your weight and reduce the risk of obesity.

CONSUMPTION: 1 medium apple

BEET APPLE SALAD

Serves 3

Prep time: 15 minutes

The crunchy apple adds fiber and sweetness to this savory salad, along with phytonutrients and antioxidants. Did you know there are more than 100 varieties of apples grown commercially in the United States? For this salad, I recommend Fuji, Honeycrisp, or Gala apples.

INGREDIENTS

2 apples, cored and cut into matchsticks

2 cooked beets, cut into matchsticks

4 celery stalks, thinly sliced

¼ cup roughly chopped walnuts

1 shallot, minced

Juice of 1 lemon

¼ cup extra-virgin olive oil

Salt

Freshly ground black pepper

2 endive heads, roughly chopped

1. In a large bowl, stir together the apples, beets, celery, walnuts, shallot, and lemon juice.

2. Drizzle the olive oil over the salad and toss to combine. Taste and season with salt and pepper.

3. Serve over a bed of chopped endive.

STORAGE TIP

Keep the beet and apple mixture separate from the endive until serving.

VARIATION TIP

This salad is delicious when mixed with a nutty whole grain, such as farro, quinoa, or barley. If you don't have (or like) walnuts, pistachios go very well in their place.

Per Serving: Calories: 393; Saturated Fat: 3g; Total Fat: 25g; Protein: 8g; Total Carbs: 43g; Fiber: 17g; Sodium: 197mg

BIRCHER MUESLI

Serves 2

Prep time: 15 minutes, plus overnight soaking

Apples are the star of this Swiss dish, which is the original overnight oats. With copious amounts of fiber and healthy fat, this breakfast will energize you (and keep you regular). Chia seeds, flaxseed, and the pectin in apples can help combat constipation.

INGREDIENTS

1 cup old-fashioned rolled oats

¾ cup unsweetened coconut milk

1 apple, cored and chopped into
  ¼-inch pieces

½ cup coconut yogurt

2 tablespoons chia seeds

2 tablespoons coconut flakes

1 tablespoon flaxseed

2 teaspoons maple syrup

¼ teaspoon ground cinnamon

In a large bowl, stir together the oats, coconut milk, apple, coconut yogurt, chia seeds, coconut flakes, flaxseed, maple syrup, and cinnamon until well combined. Cover and refrigerate overnight. Serve cold.

INGREDIENT TIP

You can use any variety of nut or plant-based milk for this recipe. The coconut yogurt adds creaminess but, if you can't find it, use any nondairy yogurt you like.

STORAGE TIP

You can make this muesli in 2 Mason jars and refrigerate them overnight for an easy grab-and-go breakfast during the week. You can use any jar or container; I use my glass nut butter jars.

Per Serving: Calories: 394; Saturated Fat: 5g; Total Fat: 13g; Protein: 10g; Total Carbs: 62g; Fiber: 14g; Sodium: 8mg

PINEAPPLES

A symbol of hospitality, the spiky tropical pineapple got its name in the seventeenth century for its resemblance to pinecones. Pineapple is most celebrated for its use as a digestive aid. If you're looking to cure an upset stomach, canned pineapple may be void of the important digestion-promoting enzyme bromelain due to the high heat used in the canning process, so fresh is best. For a sweet low-calorie, highly nutritious treat, I recommend frozen pineapple chunks.

AT A GLANCE: bromelain, manganese, potassium, vitamins B_1 and C

HEALING POWER: The enzyme bromelain helps break down proteins in food. It's interesting to note that bromelain is also used as a commercial meat tenderizer. Along with bromelain, vitamin C reduces inflammation in the body. Vitamin C acts as an antioxidant, fighting free radicals and ridding the body of unwanted toxic cells. Potassium helps regulate fluid balance and boosts the immune system. The mineral manganese is used by the body to make collagen. B vitamins, such as the vitamin B_1, or thiamin, help the body use energy effectively. Thiamin facilitates the body's use of carbohydrates for energy and is critical for glucose metabolism.

HEALTH BENEFITS/MEDICAL CONDITIONS: The bromelain content in pineapple may benefit those with various inflammatory conditions, such as asthma, and may help athletes recover more quickly after strenuous exercise. Bromelain eases inflammation, especially related to sinuses and nasal swelling. It also helps fight cancer. Pineapple may be helpful for those with lower levels of stomach acid, like the elderly or those with frequent indigestion. The complex carbohydrates found in this sweet fruit, along with vitamin B_1, can provide increased energy. The vitamin C in pineapple boosts the immune system and can help reduce the duration of a cold. The manganese found in pineapple may improve bone health and benefit those with osteoporosis.

CONSUMPTION: 1 cup cut-up pineapple

PINEAPPLE KALE SMOOTHIE

Serves 2

Prep time: 5 minutes

This tropical blend will help keep you full for hours and help move things along if you're suffering from constipation. Chia seeds and avocado are great sources of healthy fat that can help lubricate the intestines. Pineapple, with its high fiber and water content, helps promote regularity.

INGREDIENTS

1 cup frozen or fresh kale, stemmed and leaves roughly chopped

1 cup coconut water

½ cup frozen pineapple chunks

½ banana, peeled and frozen

½ avocado, peeled and pitted

1 tablespoon chia seeds

3 or 4 ice cubes

In a high-speed blender, combine the kale, coconut water, pineapple, banana, avocado, chia seeds, and ice. Blend on high speed until smooth.

INGREDIENT TIP

I recommend using frozen fruits and veggies in smoothies to get a creamier consistency. If you prefer to use fresh, decrease the amount of coconut water. Frozen fruit is picked at the peak of ripeness and is very affordable, so I stock my freezer with organic varieties.

Per Serving: Calories: 390; Saturated Fat: 2g; Total Fat: 18g; Protein: 7g; Total Carbs: 58g; Fiber: 14g; Sodium: 115mg

PINEAPPLE "NICE" CREAM

Serves 2

Prep time: 5 minutes

Nondairy pineapple ice cream that can help improve digestion? Yes, please! Pineapple contains bromelain, a digestive enzyme that helps break down proteins, making them easier for the body to absorb. Frozen pineapple cuts preparation time, is affordable, and can be found any time of year.

INGREDIENTS

2 cups frozen pineapple chunks

1 banana, peeled and frozen

½ cup unsweetened vanilla almond milk, or other nut or seed milk, plus more as needed

In a high-speed blender, combine the pineapple, banana, and coconut milk. Blend on high speed until smooth, adding more coconut milk, if needed for your desired consistency.

VARIATION TIP

Top your "nice" cream with slivered almonds, coconut flakes, cacao nibs, or crushed walnuts to add a little texture and boost nutrition even further!

Per Serving: Calories: 141; Saturated Fat: 0g; Total Fat: 1g; Protein: 2g; Total Carbs: 35g; Fiber: 4g; Sodium: 37mg

AVOCADOS

Yes, avocados are considered a fruit! The fruit fits all the botanical criteria for a berry and, like berries, avocados are incredibly nutritious and healing. The avocado tree is one of the oldest known food-producing plants in Mexico, and the Aztecs used the avocado to treat various ailments. They made a tea from the leaves to create a cough remedy and applied the leaves topically to heal bruises. The Aztecs also thought the avocado promoted fertility, and similarly, the Maya believed the fruit to be an aphrodisiac. The healthy fats in avocado can help promote fertility, and avocados are a great food for pregnant women.

AT A GLANCE: potassium, vitamins B_5 and E

HEALING POWER: Avocados are known for being low in carbohydrates and high in healthy, unsaturated fat. The fruit is considered nutrient-dense and full of healthy fats, which can promote satiety. According to the USDA, one avocado contains 975 milligrams of potassium as compared with the 422 milligrams found in one medium banana. This potassium helps regulate blood pressure and maintain fluid balance. Avocados are rich in vitamin E, which works as an antioxidant to protect tissues from free radicals. The creamy, green-hued fruit provides energy through caloric density, but also through energizing B vitamins such as vitamin B_5. Also known as pantothenic acid, vitamin B_5 is needed in the body to convert the food you eat into energy. It also helps make hormones, especially the sex and stress-related hormones in the adrenal glands.

HEALTH BENEFITS/MEDICAL CONDITIONS: The vitamin E content in avocados can help promote healthy skin and circulation. Along with other antioxidants, such as vitamins A and C, vitamin E is a powerful antioxidant that may protect against cancer. The potassium and healthy fat content in avocados may protect against heart disease. Avocados are full of fiber and low in carbohydrates, making them a great option for people with diabetes and those looking to lose weight. The B vitamin content in avocados makes them a great food for supporting hormones, especially regarding stress.

CONSUMPTION: ½ to 1 medium avocado

AVOCADO CHOCOLATE MOUSSE

Serves 2

Prep time: 10 minutes

Indulge your chocolate craving with this dairy-free mousse. This rich avocado cacao mousse is free of refined sugars, using banana and a drop of maple syrup to add sweetness. The potassium-rich treat may help promote healthy blood pressure levels.

INGREDIENTS

1 avocado, peeled, halved, and pitted

1 banana, peeled

2 tablespoons cacao powder

1 teaspoon maple syrup

¼ teaspoon ground cinnamon

1 to 2 tablespoons almond milk, plus more as needed

In a high-speed blender or food processor, combine the avocado, banana, cacao powder, maple syrup, and cinnamon. Blend until smooth, stopping to scrape down the sides, as needed. Blend in the almond milk, 1 tablespoon at a time as needed to help blend and achieve your desired consistency.

STORAGE TIP

For best taste, split the mousse between 2 bowls and serve immediately. Otherwise, keep covered and refrigerated for a maximum of 1 day.

Per Serving: Calories: 259; Saturated Fat: 4g; Total Fat: 18g; Protein: 6g; Total Carbs: 34g; Fiber: 14g; Sodium: 19mg

AVOCADO CAESAR DRESSING

Makes about 1 cup

Prep time: 5 minutes

Caesar dressing is a crowd pleaser, and it's very easy to make a plant-based version. The creaminess of avocado creates the perfect Caesar texture, and it's great for salads, grain bowls, and dipping. I recommend using the dressing to make a kale Caesar salad. Top the salad with Roasted Chickpeas (page 127) for extra crunch.

INGREDIENTS

1 ripe avocado, peeled, halved, and pitted

Juice of ½ lemon

2 garlic cloves, minced

1 tablespoon Dijon mustard

1 teaspoon salt

In a high-speed blender, combine the avocado, lemon juice, garlic, mustard, and salt. Blend until smooth, stopping to scrape down the sides, as needed. If the dressing is too thick, add water, 1 teaspoon at a time, to make blending easier.

INGREDIENT TIP

Buy an avocado a few days before you want to use it to ensure ripeness. To ripen an avocado faster, place the avocado and a banana in a loosely closed paper bag. The ethylene gas from the banana will trigger ripening in the avocado. If you want to slow the ripening process of an avocado, refrigerate it.

Per Serving (2 tablespoons): Calories: 39; Saturated Fat: 1g; Total Fat: 3g; Protein: 1g; Total Carbs: 2g; Fiber: 2g; Sodium: 315mg

BLUEBERRIES

Grown predominately in North America, the blueberry is a close relation to the super-food cranberry. Blueberries may even have the same urinary tract health benefits as the tangy cranberry. Native Americans used blueberry juice to treat coughs, and as a dye for cloth. Blueberries are now used frequently in skin care products because of its soothing, inflammation-fighting powers. I love to grab a handful of frozen wild blueberries for a sweet snack.

AT A GLANCE: anthocyanins, fiber, vitamin C

HEALING POWER: The bluish pigment gives the blueberry its name. Blueberries are one of the best food sources of antioxidants, especially anthocyanins, which are incredibly healing. As antioxidants, anthocyanins fight harmful free radicals in the body, preventing cell damage and protecting against chronic diseases and cancer. Anthocyanins have also been shown to preserve skin health and fight aging. The anthocyanins prevent oxidative damage and the high levels of vitamin C help build and rebuild collagen.

HEALTH BENEFITS/MEDICAL CONDITIONS: The antioxidants in blueberries are great for preventing sun damage, including wrinkles and age spots. Blueberries contain high amounts of water, promoting digestive health and weight loss. According to the USDA, 1 cup of blueberries contains about 4 grams of dietary fiber. This fiber is helpful for those with diabetes, as fiber helps modulate blood sugar response. The fiber in berries, especially insoluble fiber, draws water into the intestines to bulk up the stool. For this reason, blueberries may be a great solution for constipation and hemorrhoids. Anthocyanins protect against cancer, but they may also prevent cardiovascular disease and promote brain health.

CONSUMPTION: 1 cup fresh or frozen

BLUEBERRY CHIA JAM

Serves 10
Prep time: 5 minutes
Cook time: 8 minutes

Traditional jam is prepared with loads of added sugar and lacks actual nutrients. This simple recipe provides copious antioxidants from blueberries, as well as protein and healthy fat from chia seeds. Enjoy this jam in a PB&J, in a parfait, or as a whole-grain toast topper!

INGREDIENTS

1 cup frozen or fresh blueberries

2 tablespoons chia seeds

1 tablespoon freshly squeezed lemon juice

1 tablespoon maple syrup

1. In a small saucepan over low heat, warm the blueberries. Cook for about 8 minutes, stirring and mashing the blueberries into a syrup-like consistency.

2. Remove from the heat and stir in the chia seeds, lemon juice, and maple syrup. Let cool, then transfer to a glass jar, cover tightly, and refrigerate.

STORAGE TIP

This jam will last for about 2 weeks in the refrigerator.

Per Serving: Calories: 28; Saturated Fat: 0g; Total Fat: 1g; Protein: 1g; Total Carbs: 5g; Fiber: 1g; Sodium: 1mg

PB&J SMOOTHIE

Serves 1

Prep time: 5 minutes

Wild blueberries make this blend a delicious superfood treat any time of day. What's the difference between wild and regular blueberries? The wild berries are smaller, but sweeter, and have more intense flavor. The wild variety contains less water, so the berries freeze better. Note that wild isn't synonymous with organic, so check the label.

INGREDIENTS

¾ cup unsweetened plain almond milk

½ banana, peeled and frozen

½ cup frozen spinach

¼ cup frozen wild blueberries

2 tablespoons unsalted peanut butter

1 tablespoon ground flaxseed

3 or 4 ice cubes

In a high-speed blender, combine the almond milk, banana, spinach, blueberries, peanut butter, flaxseed, and ice. Blend on high speed until smooth.

VARIATION TIP

If you're not a fan of green smoothies, leave out the spinach. If you're looking for a lower-calorie option, reduce the peanut butter to 1 tablespoon.

Per Serving: Calories: 390; Saturated Fat: 12g; Total Fat: 25g; Protein: 12g; Total Carbs: 31g; Fiber: 11g; Sodium: 283mg

BANANAS

This yellow, fibrous fruit has been a solution for both diarrhea and constipation in many cultures and has even been proven to protect against stomach ulcers and heartburn. Mashed ripe banana can be used topically as a treatment for burns and wounds. The peel of the fruit has also been used in traditional and folk medicine to promote the healing of sunburns, bug bites, and minor burns. A banana peel tea is thought to improve sleep.

AT A GLANCE: fiber, potassium, vitamin B_6

HEALING POWER: The combination of fiber and complex carbohydrates in bananas provides slow-release energy. Unripe bananas have a large amount of resistant starch, a compound similar to fiber, which passes through the gut undigested and helps form beneficial bacteria. Bananas may be a good stress reliever due to their B_6 content, which is key for mood regulation. Low levels of vitamin B_6 are associated with depression, as B_6 is needed to make serotonin, the feel-good, happy hormone. B_6 also promotes optimal heart health and immunity. Bananas are known for their high potassium content, which works in the body to control blood pressure and influence bone health. Potassium is also a great electrolyte that helps maintain the body's fluid balance.

HEALTH BENEFITS/MEDICAL CONDITIONS: The B_6 levels in bananas may help reduce stress levels and help those with anxiety and insomnia. The B_6 may also improve premenstrual syndrome and reduce nausea during pregnancy. Bananas are a great source of energy for athletes, especially those who need to restore potassium and glycogen (carbohydrate stored in the muscle) levels. The potassium in bananas may promote optimal heart and bone health. The resistant starch content in bananas may help protect against colorectal cancer. Bananas are a great treatment for constipation thanks to the high soluble fiber content. Bananas can also help reduce bloating with a two-pronged approach—potassium helps the body balance fluids and fiber can help ease digestion, moving things along.

CONSUMPTION: 1 medium banana

BANANA OAT PANCAKES

Serves 2

Prep time: 20 minutes

Cook time: 10 minutes

This gluten-free recipe is a weekend favorite that can be whipped up quickly. Store-bought pancake mix typically contains processed flours, hydrogenated oils, and lots of refined sugar. Swapping your regular pancake mix for this recipe may help promote blood sugar control, encourage weight loss, and boost energy.

INGREDIENTS

6 tablespoons water

2 tablespoons ground flaxseed

2 bananas, peeled

⅔ cup old-fashioned rolled oats

½ cup unsweetened vanilla almond milk

1 teaspoon baking powder

1 teaspoon apple cider vinegar

1 teaspoon ground cinnamon

Coconut oil, for frying

1. In a small bowl, make a "flax egg" by mixing the water and flaxseed. Let sit for 10 minutes.

2. In a blender, combine the flax egg, bananas, oats, almond milk, baking powder, vinegar, and cinnamon. Blend until smooth. Let the batter sit for 5 minutes to thicken.

3. In a skillet over medium heat, melt 1 tablespoon of coconut oil. Add about ¼ cup of batter per pancake to the skillet and cook for about 3 minutes per side, or until set. Repeat with remaining batter, adding more coconut oil to the skillet, as needed.

VARIATION TIP

After blending the ingredients, add blueberries, raspberries, or any special pancake fillings you like. Serve with maple syrup, Blueberry Chia Jam (page 87), or a nut butter like the Homemade Roasted Maple Almond Butter (page 129).

Per Serving: Calories: 472; Saturated Fat: 24g; Total Fat: 34g; Protein: 6g; Total Carbs: 43g; Fiber: 9g; Sodium: 49mg

BANANA CHIA PUDDING

Serves 1

Prep time: 5 minutes, plus overnight refrigeration

Ch-ch-ch-chia! Chia seeds are small, but mighty. They're an excellent source of plant-based omega-3 fatty acids that help promote "good" cholesterol. Mixing chia seeds with banana to make this easy grab-and-go breakfast is my favorite way to enjoy the copious other nutrients of the seed, such as fiber, protein, and calcium.

INGREDIENTS

¾ cup unsweetened vanilla almond milk

½ ripe banana, peeled and mashed

2 tablespoons chia seeds

¼ teaspoon ground cinnamon

In a small bowl or airtight container, stir together the almond milk, mashed banana, chia seeds, and cinnamon. Cover and refrigerate overnight, or for at least 8 hours.

VARIATION TIP

Chia pudding can be served warm or cold. I love warm chia pudding with ½ cup blueberries mixed in. You can warm the pudding on the stove or in the microwave.

Per Serving: Calories: 222; Saturated Fat: 1g; Total Fat: 11g; Protein: 6g; Total Carbs: 27g; Fiber: 12g; Sodium: 140mg

WATERMELONS

Ancient Egyptians used watermelon to treat male reproductive issues such as prostate inflammation. Traditional Chinese medicine considers watermelon to have a cooling effect and uses the fruit to treat fluid-related diseases, such as thirst and inflammation of the urinary tract. Many medicinal uses of watermelon relate to hydration because of watermelon's high fluid content. Watermelon seeds are actually incredibly nutritious. If you choose to eat the seeds, try roasting or sprouting them.

AT A GLANCE: beta-carotene, lycopene, potassium, vitamin C

HEALING POWER: Lycopene, the carotenoid found also found in tomatoes, is an incredibly powerful antioxidant that also contributes the pink and red color to the fruit. Lycopene slows and stops the growth of cancer cells. It works by neutralizing toxic free radicals that can damage your cells. Other antioxidants in watermelon, specifically beta-carotene and vitamin C, help fight free radicals and reduce inflammation. Beta-carotene is the precursor to vitamin A, a powerful vision-promoting vitamin. Watermelon is packed with potassium and tons of water, which help promote fluid balance. The fruit's large water percentage acts as a natural diuretic and can help prevent bloating. Note that watermelon is naturally high in fructose, which is not completely absorbed in the gut, and can lead to uncomfortable bloating and gas in some people.

HEALTH BENEFITS/MEDICAL CONDITIONS: The lycopene, beta-carotene, and vitamin C found in watermelon all act as powerful antioxidants and can help prevent cancer. Lycopene is also great for skin health and helps reduce inflammation and damage to collagen in the skin. Beta-carotene and vitamin C may protect against stroke, boost the immune system, and decrease inflammation. The potassium in watermelon may promote heart health and improve nerve function. Beta-carotene promotes optimal eye health, especially countering night blindness. The hydrating water content of watermelon can help promote weight loss. The diuretic capabilities of watermelon also help relieve fluid retention.

CONSUMPTION: 1 cup cut-up watermelon

STRAWBERRY WATERMELON LIME COOLER

Serves 2

Prep time: 5 minutes

Swap this potassium-rich beverage for your typical electrolyte drink. Watermelon is incredibly hydrating and can be a great way to rehydrate after a workout, especially during the hot summer months. I enjoy this as a treat after a long training run and add a pinch salt to help my body hold on to the water and replace lost sodium.

INGREDIENTS

1 cup cubed seedless watermelon

1 cup frozen strawberries

½ cup water

Juice of 1 lime

Pinch salt (optional)

In a high-speed blender, combine the watermelon, strawberries, water, lime juice, and salt (if using). Blend on high speed until smooth.

VARIATION TIP

This recipe makes delicious ice pops. Pour any extra beverage into an ice pop mold and freeze for a hydrating frozen treat.

Per Serving: Calories: 56; Saturated Fat: 0g; Total Fat: 0g; Protein: 1g; Total Carbs: 15g; Fiber: 3g; Sodium: 2mg

WATERMELON, TOMATO, AND RED ONION SALAD

Serves 5

Prep time: 10 minutes, plus 2 hours to marinate (optional)

The vibrant red color of this salad screams lycopene! Lycopene, the red pigment and antioxidant found in the watermelon, tomatoes, and red onion, may improve heart health. Red onion also contains the antioxidant quercetin. Don't be too quick to shed the outer layers of the red onion, as research shows that quercetin levels are highest in the outer rings.

INGREDIENTS

5 cups seedless (½-inch) watermelon cubes

1½ pounds ripe tomatoes, cut into
  ½-inch cubes

1 small red onion, quartered and thinly sliced

½ cup red wine vinegar

¼ cup extra-virgin olive oil

Salt

Freshly ground black pepper

In a large bowl, combine the watermelon and tomatoes. Add the red onion, vinegar, and olive oil. Mix well. Season with salt and pepper. Serve immediately, or cover, refrigerate, and let marinate for 2 hours, if desired.

INGREDIENT TIP

Buy pre-cut watermelon to reduce prep time substantially.

Per Serving: Calories: 167; Saturated Fat: 2g; Total Fat: 11g; Protein: 2g; Total Carbs: 18g; Fiber: 3g; Sodium: 41mg

POMEGRANATES

For thousands of years, the pomegranate has been a symbol of prosperity and hope, as well as fertility. The rind of the pomegranate has been used in Ayurvedic practice as a remedy for digestive distress. The bitter seeds (arils) and juice are thought to balance a diet high in sweet and fatty foods. Pomegranates can be challenging to eat because of the messy seeds.

AT A GLANCE: ellagitannin, fiber, punicic acid

HEALING POWER: Pomegranate juice has been shown to have antioxidant activity that's three times higher than red wine or green tea. Pomegranates contain various types of antioxidants, one of which is punicic acid, which has been shown to decrease cholesterol and triglyceride levels. It helps prevent atherosclerosis, or the buildup of plaque in the artery walls. The antioxidants in pomegranates also protect against prostate cancer by inhibiting cell growth and inducing apoptosis, or cell death. One cancer-fighting phytochemical in pomegranates, known as ellagitannin, is metabolized in the intestine and works to inhibit prostate cancer cell growth.

HEALTH BENEFITS/MEDICAL CONDITIONS: Pomegranates are rich in antioxidants that help protect against various cancers, including breast, lung, skin, and colon cancers. The antioxidant power of pomegranates may preserve and protect prostate health. Phytochemicals in pomegranates promote cardiovascular health and function. According to the USDA, 1 cup of pomegranate arils contains 3.5 grams of dietary fiber. This fiber content may help promote weight loss, normalize bowel habits, control blood sugar levels, and even lower cholesterol levels. New research suggests that pomegranate juice may help prevent pregnancy complications, echoing the historical use of the food.

CONSUMPTION: ½ cup pomegranate arils

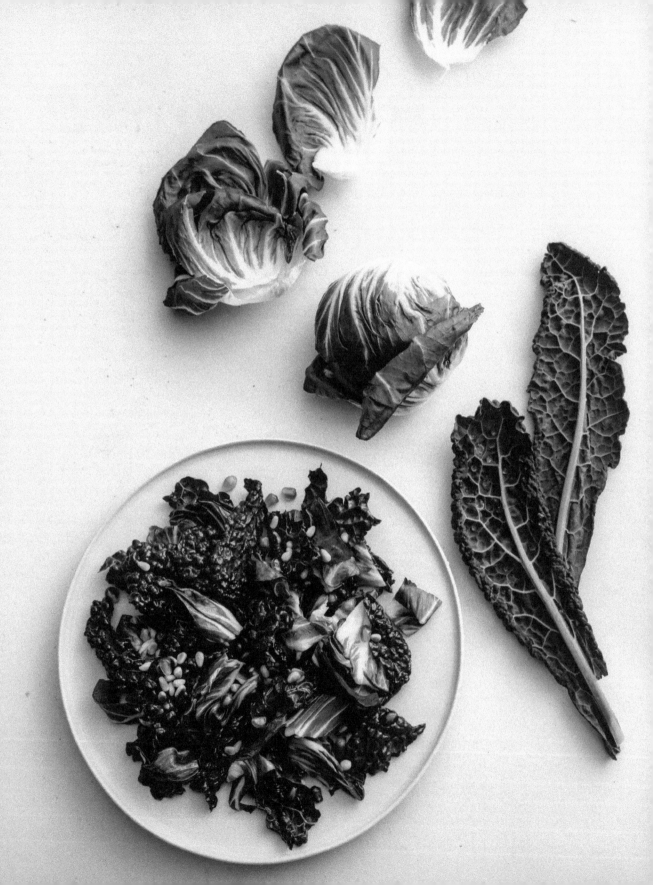

KALE AND RADICCHIO SALAD
WITH POMEGRANATE

Serves 4

Prep time: 15 minutes

Invite me to a party and this is probably what I'll bring! A trick to always having a healthy party option available is to offer to bring a salad. This particular salad is full of fiber and antioxidant-rich veggies as well as healthy fats. If you're working with a thicker variety of kale, I recommend adding the vinaigrette and massaging it into the kale before you get to the party. For baby kale, add the dressing just before serving.

INGREDIENTS

2 bunches lacinato, Tuscan, or dinosaur kale, stemmed, leaves torn into small pieces

1 radicchio head, roughly chopped

¼ cup Classic Lemon Apple Cider Vinaigrette (page 76)

1 cup pomegranate arils

¼ cup pine nuts, toasted (optional)

In a large bowl, combine the kale and radicchio. Add the vinaigrette and toss well to combine. Top with the pomegranate arils and pine nuts (if using) and serve.

STORAGE TIP

This salad keeps fairly well, so you can refrigerate leftovers to enjoy the next day.

INGREDIENT TIP

If traditional kale is tough on your stomach, try baby kale, which may be easier to digest.

Per Serving: Calories: 189; Saturated Fat: 1g; Total Fat: 4g; Protein: 6g; Total Carbs: 34g; Fiber: 4g; Sodium: 128mg

POMEGRANATE PARFAIT

Serves 1

Prep time: 5 minutes

Pomegranate and pumpkin seeds are a smart swap for sugary granola in a parfait. The red, juicy arils boost fiber and antioxidant content and pumpkin seeds are a great source of plant-based iron. When choosing a nondairy yogurt, look for a short ingredient list without extra sugar.

INGREDIENTS

1 cup nondairy yogurt (almond, coconut, cashew, etc.), divided

½ cup pomegranate arils, divided

2 tablespoons pumpkin seeds

In a small glass jar or bowl, place ½ cup of yogurt. Top with ¼ cup of pomegranate arils. Layer on the remaining ½ cup of yogurt and remaining ¼ cup pomegranate arils. Sprinkle the pumpkin seeds over the top.

INGREDIENT TIP

To seed a pomegranate without all the mess, cut the pomegranate in half. Submerge half of the pomegranate in a large bowl filled with cold water. Use your fingers to free the arils and remove the white pith. Repeat with the second half, drain the water, and reserve the arils.

Per Serving: Calories: 314; Saturated Fat: 8g; Total Fat: 18g; Protein: 8g; Total Carbs: 34g; Fiber: 2g; Sodium: 47mg

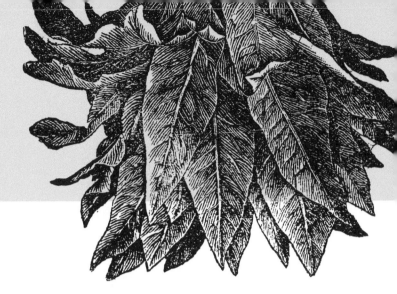

HOW TO NATURALLY ACCELERATE (OR SLOW) FRUIT RIPENING

Need to ripen an avocado or pear? Look no further than your fruit bowl. Bananas give off ethylene gas, which can help speed ripening in other fruits. This naturally occurring, scent-free gas acts as a plant hormone, promoting other plants' development. When a fruit is exposed to ethylene, the acids in the fruit begin to break down and the fruit becomes softer. You can further accelerate ripening by trapping the ethylene gas by placing the unripe fruit and a banana in a paper bag. Do you need a few more days before you use the fruit? Slow the ripening process by placing the fruit in the refrigerator.

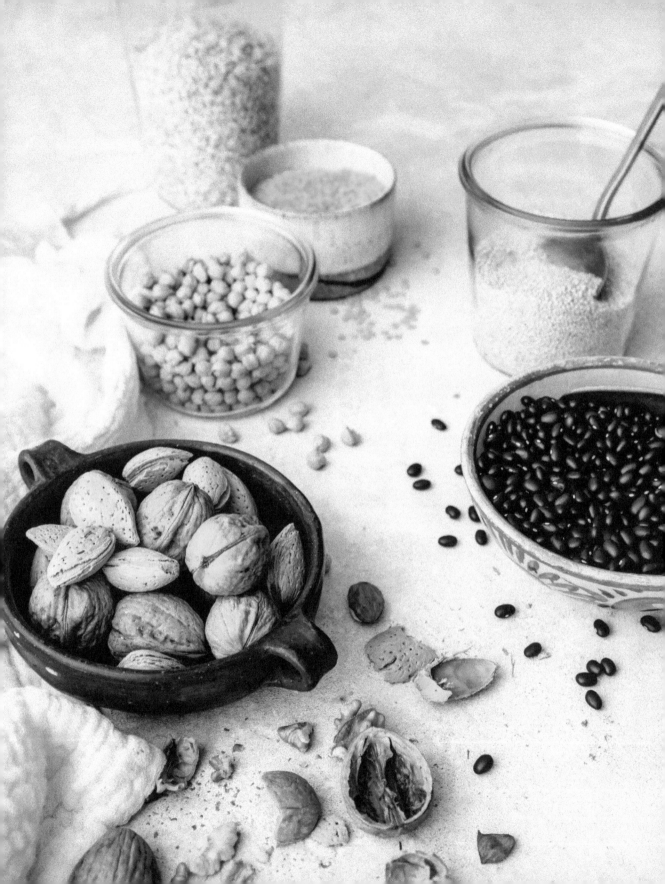

5

Whole Grains, Legumes, and Nuts

By now, you've likely heard you should make half your grains "whole," but do you know what that means? Grains are considered "whole grains" when they are the entire seed of a plant. During processing, the outer layers of the seed (the bran and germ) are removed. Thus, refined grains are made up only of the remaining starchy endosperm. Whole grains provide more protein, vitamins, minerals, and fiber than their processed counterparts. Like whole grains, legumes—such as beans, peas, and lentils—are incredibly rich in protein and fiber and have remarkable healing powers. In this chapter, I highlight 10 healing whole grains, legumes, and nuts and offer delicious, easy ways to reap their various benefits.

BROWN RICE

In traditional Chinese medicine, rice is thought to strengthen the life force (or the energizing *qi*) and promote digestion. Congee, a starchy Chinese rice soup, has been used as a digestive aid for centuries. Brown rice is an easy swap for white rice, but many clients ask why it's nutritionally superior. The processing of brown rice removes only the hull of the rice kernel, whereas the milling and polishing that occurs when brown rice is further refined to white rice destroys many of its B vitamins, iron, and fiber.

AT A GLANCE: fiber, manganese, selenium

HEALING POWER: This naturally gluten-free grain improves digestive function with its high fiber content. Fiber works in the bowels to remove waste and alleviate constipation. Although brown rice takes longer than white rice to break down because of its fiber content, it is gentle on the stomach with its high amounts of complex carbohydrates. These slow-burning carbohydrates can quell an uneasy stomach and are absorbed more easily than protein and fats. Brown rice contains various healing nutrients such as selenium, iron, and B vitamins. Selenium helps fight cancer by repairing damaged cells and inhibiting the growth of cancer cells. Like selenium, the mineral manganese plays an anti-oxidative role, helping fight cancer and promote energy production.

HEALTH BENEFITS/MEDICAL CONDITIONS: The fiber in brown rice helps lower cholesterol and is beneficial to heart health. Brown rice is considered a low-calorie, low-glycemic food, meaning it will not raise blood sugar quickly after consuming it, so it is good for people with diabetes. The high fiber content in brown rice benefits digestive health and those seeking to lose weight. Selenium in brown rice promotes optimal thyroid health. The antioxidant functions of selenium and manganese in the body help protect against cancer.

CONSUMPTION: 1 cup cooked brown rice

SAVORY SHALLOT BROWN RICE

Serves 3
Prep time: 5 minutes
Cook time: 50 minutes

Caramelized shallots and vegetable broth bring regular brown rice to the next flavor level. Brown rice is a great side dish or base to any veggie-based meal, but sometimes requires a bit more salt for flavoring than is ideal to use. Infusing the rice with a low-sodium broth and the sweet, subtle flavor of shallot provides that flavor in a healthier way.

INGREDIENTS

1 tablespoon extra-virgin olive oil

1 shallot, very thinly sliced

1 cup brown rice

2 cups low-sodium vegetable broth

1 bay leaf

Salt

Freshly ground black pepper

1. In a small saucepan over medium-low heat, heat the olive oil. Add the shallot and cook for about 2 minutes until soft and starting to brown.

2. Add the rice, vegetable broth, and bay leaf to the saucepan and bring the liquid to a boil. Reduce the heat to low, cover the pan, and cook for 45 minutes.

3. Remove the rice from the heat, remove the lid, and stir the rice. Re-cover the pan and let stand for 10 minutes. Remove the bay leaf and discard. Use a fork to fluff the rice, then serve warm.

COOKING TIP

If the liquid is not fully absorbed after 45 minutes, cook the rice for another 5 to 10 minutes, watching so it doesn't burn.

STORAGE TIP

Refrigerate cooked brown rice in an airtight container for 3 to 5 days, or freeze it for up to 3 months.

Per Serving: Calories: 282; Saturated Fat: 1g; Total Fat: 6g; Protein: 6g; Total Carbs: 50g; Fiber: 2g; Sodium: 100mg

BROWN RICE BOWL WITH CREAMY LIME DRESSING

Serves 1

Prep time: 5 minutes

Brown rice bowls are one of my staples for lunch or dinner. The combination of brown rice and black beans tastes delicious, but is also extra nutritious because the two complementary foods combine to create a complete protein. What's a complete protein? It means it contains all the essential amino acids our bodies need.

INGREDIENTS

1 cup Savory Shallot Brown Rice (page 103)

1 cup cooked black beans

½ avocado, peeled, pitted, and cut lengthwise into slices

1 tomato, chopped

2 tablespoons Creamy Lime Dressing (page 164)

2 tablespoons roughly chopped fresh cilantro (optional)

Place the brown rice in a bowl. Top with the black beans, avocado, and tomato. Drizzle the dressing on top and sprinkle with cilantro (if using).

COOKING TIP

Don't have time to make the brown rice or black beans from scratch? Purchase pre-cooked, canned, frozen, or shelf-stable packaged organic black beans and brown rice.

Per Serving: Calories: 707; Saturated Fat: 5g; Total Fat: 34g; Protein: 22g; Total Carbs: 86g; Fiber: 25g; Sodium: 44mg

OATS

Oats are widely used to soothe internal and external concerns. Oats are a key ingredient in various cosmetics, including sensitive skin lotions. Oat baths are a quick way to get relief from chicken pox and poison ivy. As a food source, oats are deeply woven into many cultures. Porridge and gruel made from oats are key breakfast foods in Scotland. Today, oats are promoted as a heart-healthy breakfast option by the American Heart Association.

AT A GLANCE: avenanthramide, fiber, melatonin, saponins

HEALING POWER: Oats are a heart-healthy food thanks to their high content of a soluble fiber known as beta-glucans. Beta-glucans help remove cholesterol from the body by binding with the bad cholesterol, then eliminating it through digestion. This process prevents the cholesterol from clogging arteries. Oats also contain a unique antioxidant, avenanthramide, that protects against cancer and heart disease. This versatile grain is considered a good source of melatonin, a hormone that can promote sleep. Topically, oats are great for helping relieve dry skin because of their natural cleaning powers from a compound called saponins.

HEALTH BENEFITS/MEDICAL CONDITIONS: The soluble fiber in oats reduces the risk of heart disease and atherosclerosis by reducing cholesterol and blood pressure, and may help lower blood sugar, making oats a good food for people with diabetes. Oats are naturally gluten free, although people with celiac disease or other gluten sensitivities must carefully check packaging to ensure the oats are produced in a gluten-free facility. Whole grains, including oats, may help decrease the incidences of digestive diseases and colorectal cancer. Oats may promote good sleep and prevent insomnia. Oats may benefit skin, especially acne. Oats are known to act as a galactagogue, which supports lactating women.

CONSUMPTION: ½ cup uncooked, or 1 cup cooked

NO-BAKE ENERGY BITES

Makes 16 to 20 bites

Prep time: 10 minutes

If you're looking for an ideal snack, look no further. Full of complex carbohydrates, healthy fats, and plant-based proteins, these simple bites are the perfect sweet treat. You can make your own variations on the recipe and include various items such as goji berries or dried blueberries for an extra antioxidant boost.

INGREDIENTS

2 cups old-fashioned rolled oats

1 cup nut butter, or seed butter

½ cup ground flaxseed

⅓ cup maple syrup, or honey

⅓ cup dark chocolate chips (at least 70 percent cacao)

¼ cup chia seeds

¼ cup coconut flakes

1 teaspoon vanilla extract

1. In a large bowl, stir together the oats, nut butter, flaxseed, maple syrup, chocolate chips, chia seeds, coconut flakes, and vanilla until well combined.

2. Roll the oat mixture into 1-inch balls. Refrigerate in an airtight container for 1 week, or freeze for 1 month.

VARIATION TIP

Know someone who is breastfeeding? Make these into powerful lactation bites by adding 3 tablespoons of brewer's yeast to the mix.

Per Serving (1 bite): Calories: 217; Saturated Fat: 3g; Total Fat: 13g; Protein: 6g; Total Carbs: 21g; Fiber: 4g; Sodium: 5mg

OVERNIGHT OATS

Serves 2

Prep time: 5 minutes, plus overnight refrigeration

In my opinion, breakfast really is the most important meal of the day. Start your day off right with a balanced meal like overnight oats, which has the perfect balance of protein, healthy fats, and carbs. Create your own versions by adding other superfood ingredients such as cacao, almond butter, or matcha powder. The options are endless!

INGREDIENTS

1 banana, peeled

1½ cups unsweetened plain almond milk

1 cup old-fashioned rolled oats

¼ cup chia seeds

1 teaspoon ground cinnamon

½ teaspoon vanilla extract

½ cup fresh blueberries (optional)

1. In a medium bowl, using a fork, mash the banana.

2. Stir in the almond milk, oats, chia seeds, cinnamon, and vanilla.

3. Add the blueberries (if using) and stir to combine. Cover and refrigerate overnight.

COOKING TIP

I often make a version of these overnight oats in individual Mason jars. If you're looking for a super-quick grab-and-go breakfast, mash ½ banana in a jar. Add ¾ cup almond milk, ½ cup oats, 2 tablespoons chia seeds, and a sprinkle of cinnamon. Seal the lid and shake to combine. Refrigerate overnight.

Per Serving: Calories: 428; Saturated Fat: 2g; Total Fat: 16g; Protein: 13g; Total Carbs: 59g; Fiber: 18g; Sodium: 278mg

QUINOA

Quinoa is a seed or pseudo-grain, which is naturally gluten free, high in protein, and full of fiber. It comes in various colors and is celebrated for its status as a complete protein. Quinoa is one of the few plant foods that contains all nine essential amino acids our bodies need, making it a fabulous source of plant-based protein. Indigenous to South America, the Andean people used quinoa to make a paste to heal broken bones. The Incas referred to quinoa as *chisaya mama*, or the mother of all grains.

AT A GLANCE: fiber, lignans, magnesium, omega-3 fatty acids

HEALING POWER: The magnesium in quinoa acts as a natural relaxant. It improves blood flow and can help nerve function in the body. Quinoa is rich in heart-healthy omega-3 fats, such as oleic acid and alpha-linolenic acid. These fats can help reduce inflammation and sustain energy for longer periods. Research suggests that quinoa is also a great gut health booster, as it contains prebiotics—the food for probiotics. Quinoa contains potent free radical–fighting antioxidants like quercetin. It also contains the phytoestrogen lignin, which works to stop cancer growth and development.

HEALTH BENEFITS/MEDICAL CONDITIONS: As a complete protein, quinoa is a great protein source for vegans, vegetarians, and those seeking to consume a more plant-based diet. Quinoa is full of fiber that can protect against digestive diseases and promote optimal digestion. The prebiotic content of quinoa improves gut bacteria. Fiber can also reduce the risk of many chronic diseases, including cancer. Lignans found in quinoa may protect against hormone-related cancers, such as breast cancer. The fiber and protein content of quinoa may promote weight loss. Quinoa contains bone-building components, such as magnesium and potassium, which can help prevent osteoporosis.

CONSUMPTION: 1 cup cooked quinoa

CACAO QUINOA GRANOLA

Serves 6

Prep time: 5 minutes

Cook time: 20 minutes

Take granola to the next nutritional level with cacao and quinoa. Typical granola is high in sugar and fairly low in nutrients. This recipe creates a delicious (and incredibly nutritious) blend by eliminating processed sugars and adding the health benefits from superfoods such as quinoa, nuts, and cacao nibs.

INGREDIENTS

1 cup old-fashioned rolled oats

1 cup roughly chopped almonds

1 cup roughly chopped walnuts

½ cup uncooked quinoa, any color

½ cup shelled roasted pistachios

¼ cup cacao powder

1 tablespoon ground cinnamon

¼ cup coconut oil, melted

¼ cup maple syrup

¼ cup cacao nibs

1. Preheat the oven to 350°F.

2. In a large bowl, stir together the oats, almonds, walnuts, quinoa, pistachios, cacao powder, and cinnamon.

3. In a small bowl, whisk the melted coconut oil and maple syrup to blend and immediately pour it over the dry ingredients. Mix well, then spread the granola in an even layer on a baking sheet.

4. Bake for 15 to 20 minutes, or until golden, stirring every 5 minutes to promote even browning.

5. Let cool. Mix in the cacao nibs. Keep stored in an airtight container for up to a week.

INGREDIENT TIP

Cocoa powder and cacao powder are not the same. Cocoa powder is the roasted version of cacao powder, which reduces the enzyme content of the raw cacao. Dutch-processed cocoa powder is processed once more in a potassium solution that reduces the acidity and gives it a more neural flavor. I recommend using Navitas Organics cacao powder.

Per Serving: Calories: 576; Saturated Fat: 13g; Total Fat: 42g; Protein: 17g; Total Carbs: 48g; Fiber: 14g; Sodium: 56mg

SIMPLE QUINOA SALAD

Serves 2
Prep time: 10 minutes
Cook time: 15 minutes

When my clients want a simple, protein-packed lunch or dinner, this is my first recommendation. There's nothing better than a simple "throw-together" meal made of crunchy, fresh ingredients. This colorful quinoa salad comes together easily and is bursting with flavor.

INGREDIENTS

⅔ cup uncooked quinoa, rinsed

1⅓ cups water

1 cucumber, finely chopped

1 cup halved cherry tomatoes

½ red onion, finely chopped

¼ cup chopped fresh basil

¼ cup Classic Lemon Apple Cider Vinaigrette (page 76)

Salt

Freshly ground black pepper

1. In a small saucepan over high heat, combine the quinoa and water. Bring to a boil. Once boiling, reduce the heat to low, cover the pan, and simmer for 15 minutes, or until all the liquid is absorbed. Fluff the quinoa with a fork and set aside to cool.

2. In a large bowl, combine the cooled quinoa, cucumber, tomatoes, red onion, and basil.

3. Add the vinaigrette and toss to combine the ingredients. Taste and season with salt and pepper.

INGREDIENT TIP

There are more than 100 varieties of quinoa, and they are all nutritious options. The most widely available varieties are red, white, and black. Red quinoa is best to use in salads, as it tends to hold its shape better than the other colors. Rinse quinoa before cooking to remove the natural coating, which is called saponin. This coating sometimes tastes bitter or soapy. Most boxed quinoa is pre-rinsed, but it's a good idea to give it an extra rinse in a fine-mesh sieve.

Per Serving: Calories: 353; Saturated Fat: 2g; Total Fat: 13g; Protein: 10g; Total Carbs: 53g; Fiber: 6g; Sodium: 77mg

CORN

Corn, also known as maize, is one of the most popular foods in the world and is widely used for fuel and animal feed. The Native Americans and Chinese historically used corn silk, the thread-like strands we usually discard, to treat urinary disorders. It's a controversial grain (and vegetable), as it can be highly processed and made into unhealthy items such as corn syrup. Although processed corn products are not health-promoting, unprocessed sweet corn can be a very nutritious and healing whole-grain option.

AT A GLANCE: B vitamins, carotenoids, fiber

HEALING POWER: Corn gets a bad rap for its high carbohydrate content, which is known to raise blood sugar levels; however, corn also contains a high level of fiber that helps modulate the blood sugar response. The majority of fiber in corn is insoluble, which is why corn kernels can pass through the digestive system whole. The fiber-rich complex carbohydrates can help regulate the digestive system and alleviate stomach woes. Corn contains many energy-promoting B vitamins, including folate. The carotenoids zeaxanthin and lutein give corn its yellow color. These pigments act as antioxidants in the body, helping rid the body of toxic substances like free radicals.

HEALTH BENEFITS/MEDICAL CONDITIONS: Corn may promote eye health thanks to the lutein and zeaxanthin content. These antioxidants may also help reduce inflammation in the body, support the immune system, and prevent cancer. The fiber in corn may help prevent diverticulosis and digestive issues. The B vitamins and complex carbohydrates in corn provide ample energy, making corn an optimal fuel for athletes. Pregnant women may benefit from folate, which helps prevent birth defects related to the baby's brain and spine, and may lower the risk of preeclampsia. Corn is naturally gluten free and is a good whole-grain option for those with celiac disease or gluten sensitivity.

CONSUMPTION: 1 ear corn, 1 cup cooked corn, or 3 cups popped corn

STOVETOP POPCORN

Makes 10 cups

Prep time: 5 minutes

Cook time: 5 minutes

Pop, pop, pop! My mom is a popcorn lover, and we always have it at home. Even though there are packaged options available, I love making my own and am always seeking to make it in more nutritious and delicious ways. Plus, when you make it at home it's much more affordable and it's always super crunchy.

INGREDIENTS

3 tablespoons coconut oil

½ cup popcorn kernels

Pinch sea salt (For other flavors, see Variation Tip)

1. In a large pot over medium-high heat, melt the coconut oil.

2. Add 3 popcorn kernels and cover the pot. When 1 or more kernels pop, add the remaining kernels and re-cover the pot.

3. Cook for 4 to 5 minutes, gently shaking the pot over the heat every 20 seconds to prevent the kernels from burning. The popcorn will be done when you can't hear anymore popping.

4. Turn off the heat and remove the pot from the burner. Add salt and serve.

VARIATION TIP

Try Cinnamon-Spiced Popcorn using 1 teaspoon ground cinnamon and 1 teaspoon ground ginger. Make Garlic and Herb Popcorn with 1 teaspoon garlic powder, 1 teaspoon dried rosemary, and 1 teaspoon sea salt. Try "Cheesy" Popcorn with 2 tablespoons nutritional yeast and 1 teaspoon sea salt.

Per Serving (2 cups): Calories: 159; Saturated Fat: 7g; Total Fat: 9g; Protein: 3g; Total Carbs: 21g; Fiber: 6g; Sodium: 0mg

CORN, TOMATO, AND AVOCADO SALAD

Serves 2

Prep time: 10 minutes

Cook time: 5 minutes

For me, this salad screams summer! It combines everything fresh from the farmers' market—corn, onion, basil, and tomato. The steamed corn adds sweetness, and the whole salad can be enjoyed warm. You can use raw corn, but make sure it's freshly picked for optimal sweetness and easier digestion.

INGREDIENTS

2 ears corn, husked

1 cup halved cherry tomatoes

1 avocado, peeled, halved, pitted, and cut into ½-inch chunks

2 tablespoons finely chopped red onion

2 tablespoons freshly squeezed lemon juice

1 tablespoon extra-virgin olive oil

Salt

Freshly ground black pepper

2 tablespoons roughly chopped fresh basil

COOKING TIP

To microwave-steam the corn kernels, cut the kernels off the cob and put them in a microwave-safe bowl. Add 2 tablespoons water. Cover the bowl with plastic wrap and microwave for 4 minutes. Drain the corn.

1. Place a vegetable steamer in a large pot and add enough water so the base of the pot is filled, but water is not touching the steamer. Bring the water to a boil over high heat. Break the corn ears in half and place them in the steamer. Cover the pot and cook the corn for 5 minutes. Remove the corn from the pot, let cool.

2. Cut the kernels off the cobs: Place a small bowl upside-down inside a large bowl. Stand the corn on top of the smaller bowl and, using a sharp knife, cut the corn kernels off the cob from top to bottom. The kernels will collect in the bottom of the larger bowl.

3. To the corn, add the tomatoes, avocado, red onion, lemon juice, and olive oil. Season with salt and pepper. Toss to combine and serve topped with basil.

Per Serving: Calories: 292; Saturated Fat: 3g; Total Fat: 22g; Protein: 5g; Total Carbs: 26g; Fiber: 9g; Sodium: 103mg

FARRO

Soft, chewy farro is an ancient whole grain known for its nutty, earthy flavor. Farro is most commonly found as emmer wheat, which was a keystone of the ancient Romans' diet. It's also found as einkorn and spelt. The grain is consumed across the globe and is celebrated for its various healing properties. In Ethiopia, emmer wheat is thought to help heal broken bones and is used to help mothers recover after childbirth. This Mediterranean wheat-containing grain is delicious is in soups, salads, and even as a breakfast grain.

AT A GLANCE: fiber, magnesium, niacin, selenium, zinc

HEALING POWER: Farro is a great digestive aid, as it is full of fiber, particularly resistant starch. Resistant starch isn't fully broken down in the digestive tract and converted into sugar for energy like regular starches. Instead, it is turned into short-chain fatty acids and used as a food source for bacteria in the digestive tract. The other forms of fiber, soluble and insoluble fiber, help bulk the stool and alleviate any issues pertaining to constipation. The zinc in farro promotes optimal carbohydrate digestion, as well as wound healing and improved immunity. Farro is a good whole-grain source of protein and combines with beans or legumes to form a whole protein. Farro contains components such as phenolic antioxidants and selenium that can fight free radicals.

HEALTH BENEFITS/MEDICAL CONDITIONS: The high fiber content in farro can help promote optimal heart health and may be beneficial for those with type 2 diabetes. High-fiber foods, like the whole grain farro, may help promote weight loss. Resistant starch in farro promotes good gut health, improves immunity, and may fight cancer. Note that farro contains wheat and is not gluten free, so it is not suitable for those with celiac disease or other gluten sensitivities. The magnesium in farro supports healthy nerve and muscle function. Because of the magnesium content and the complex carbohydrates that can balance blood sugar, farro may be good for headaches.

CONSUMPTION: 1 cup cooked farro

FARRO SALAD WITH FENNEL AND RAISINS

Serves 6

Prep time: 5 minutes, plus overnight soaking

Cook time: 10 minutes

This delicious grain salad is equally hearty and light. The farro provides a whole-grain base brightened with crunchy fennel and sweet raisins. The vitamin C in fennel promotes absorption of the iron content from farro and raisins. What a delicious nutrition boost!

INGREDIENTS

1 cup whole-grain farro

2½ cups water, plus more for soaking the farro

1 fennel bulb, cored and thinly sliced

1 radicchio head, cored and thinly chopped

½ cup golden raisins

¼ cup extra-virgin olive oil

1 shallot, minced

2 tablespoons freshly squeezed lemon juice

2 teaspoons honey

Salt

Freshly ground black pepper

1. Place the farro in a bowl and cover it with water. Cover the bowl and soak the farro overnight in the refrigerator. Drain the farro.

2. In a small pot over high heat, combine 2½ cups fresh water and soaked farro. Bring to a boil. Stir, reduce the heat to a simmer, and cook the farro for about 10 minutes, uncovered, until tender. Drain the farro and transfer it to a large bowl.

3. Add the fennel, radicchio, and raisins.

4. In a small bowl, whisk the olive oil, shallot, lemon juice, and honey to blend. Drizzle the dressing over the farro and toss well to combine. Taste and season with salt and pepper.

VARIATION TIP

Substitute ½ cup currants or regular sundried raisins for the golden raisins. Currants are one of my favorite dried fruits, but they can be a bit more expensive and difficult to find.

Per Serving: Calories: 287; Saturated Fat: 1g; Total Fat: 10g; Protein: 7g; Total Carbs: 44g; Fiber: 7g; Sodium: 53mg

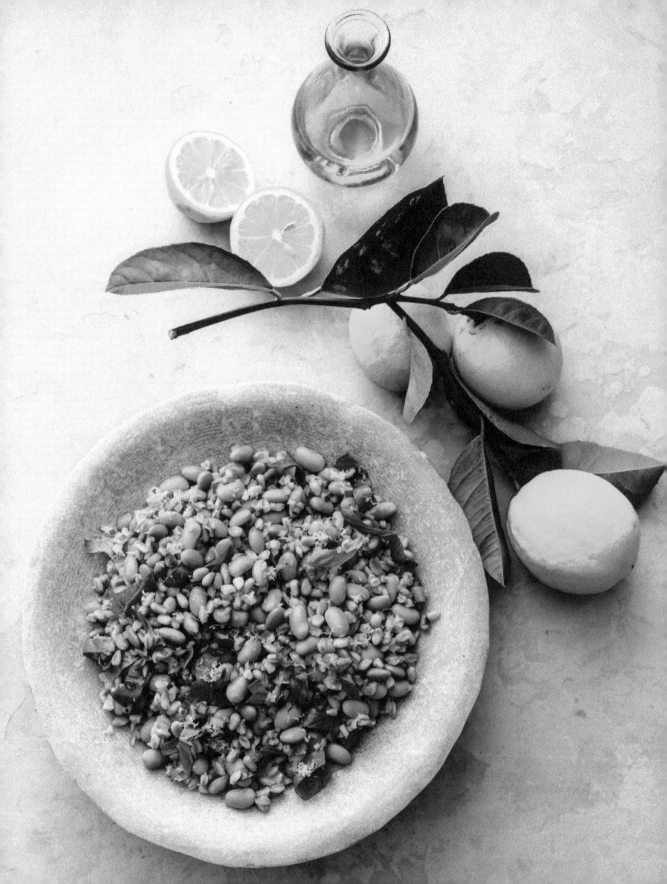

FARRO SALAD WITH EDAMAME AND PINE NUTS

Serves 4

Prep time: 10 minutes, plus overnight soaking

Cook time: 15 minutes

Complement the nutty taste of farro by combining it with soybeans, or edamame. This delicious dish is full of protein, healthy fats, and whole grains, so it is sure to keep you feeling satiated. If you've prepared the farro in advance, this meal will come together quickly and is great for a hearty plant-based dinner, with ample leftovers for lunch the next day.

INGREDIENTS

½ cup whole-grain farro

1½ cups water, plus more for soaking the farro

½ cup pine nuts

2 cups frozen shelled edamame, thawed

½ cup chopped fresh basil

¼ cup finely chopped red onion

¼ cup extra-virgin olive oil

Juice of 1 lemon

1 tablespoon grated lemon zest

Salt

Freshly ground black pepper

1. Place the farro in a bowl and cover it with water. Cover the bowl and soak the farro overnight in the refrigerator. Drain the farro.

2. In a small pot over high heat, combine 1½ cups of water and soaked farro. Bring to a boil. Stir, reduce the heat to a simmer, and cook the farro for about 10 minutes, uncovered, until tender. Drain the farro and transfer it to a large bowl. Set aside.

3. In a dry skillet over medium heat, toast the pine nuts for about 2 minutes until fragrant and lightly browned. Add them to the bowl with the farro, along with the edamame, basil, and red onion.

4. In a small bowl, whisk the olive oil, lemon juice, and lemon zest to blend. Pour the dressing over the farro and toss well to combine. Taste and season with salt and pepper.

CONTINUED

COOKING TIP

Cooking times for farro vary based on the type of farro used. This recipe uses whole-grain farro. Pearled farro will have a shorter cooking time. If you're unsure what type of farro you have, cook the grain according to the package instructions.

INGREDIENT TIP

Frozen edamame is parboiled to preserve freshness, so you don't need to cook it. Thawing it, then mixing it with a hot grain helps cook it a bit more. If you choose to heat it, you can microwave it for 2 to 3 minutes before mixing it into the salad.

Per Serving: Calories: 394; Saturated Fat: 3g; Total Fat: 27g; Protein: 11g; Total Carbs: 29g; Fiber: 7g; Sodium: 57mg

LENTILS

Lentils are a high-fiber, nutrient-dense legume with ample "slow-release" carbohydrates and protein. They come in a variety of colors, and each color has a slightly different taste and property. Red and yellow lentils are the sweetest and nuttiest-tasting lentils and are generally used in soups, curries, or dal, a traditional Indian dish. Green lentils are known for their robust flavor and are traditionally used in salads, as they retain their shape well when cooked. The highly popular brown lentil is known for its earthy flavor and a texture that holds up well in stews. Black lentils are actually the most nutritious variety, thanks to their protein, calcium, and iron content, but also the high levels of anthocyanins.

AT A GLANCE: fiber, folate, iron

HEALING POWER: With 18 grams of protein per cup, lentils are one of the most significant plant-based sources of protein, and when paired with complementary grains, they form a complete protein. Lentils contain both insoluble and soluble fiber, which absorbs water in the stomach, expands, and keeps you feeling fuller longer. For this reason, they are a great digestive aid, and also fight many chronic diseases. Part of the soluble fiber in lentils is prebiotic fiber, which is the food for gut-friendly probiotics. Probiotics also help improve digestion and immunity. If you have trouble reaping the benefits of lentils because of indigestion, consider soaking the lentils with a piece of kombu (a mineral-packed seaweed) before cooking. Soaking the lentils with kombu helps reduce the gas-producing properties of the legume.

HEALTH BENEFITS/MEDICAL CONDITIONS: The high fiber content of lentils helps control blood sugar and may be good for people with diabetes. Fiber also helps lower cholesterol and may promote optimal heart health. Fiber helps improve digestion, especially with regard to bulking stool and fighting constipation. The anti-inflammatory properties of lentils are beneficial to those with arthritis and inflammatory diseases. The iron in lentils helps prevent anemia and fatigue. Iron is critical for expectant mothers, as is folate, which helps prevent neural tube defects in the infant.

CONSUMPTION: 1 cup cooked lentils

SIMPLE LENTIL SALAD

Serves 2

Prep time: 10 minutes

Like the Simple Quinoa Salad (page 110), this dish comes together quickly and is packed with flavor and energy-sustaining nutrients. Lentils remind me of a summer spent studying in the south of France, where cold lentil salads are as common as crusty French bread. The basil and chives brighten the dish, but you can modify the flavors as you like. See the Variation Tip for ideas.

INGREDIENTS

1 (15-ounce) can no-salt-added cooked lentils, drained and rinsed

1 cup halved cherry tomatoes

¼ cup Classic Lemon Apple Cider Vinaigrette (page 76) or Roasted Garlic Dressing (page 144)

2 tablespoons chopped fresh chives

2 tablespoons chopped fresh basil

In a large bowl, toss together the lentils, cherry tomatoes, vinaigrette, chives, and basil to combine.

VARIATION TIP

Add any chopped vegetables you have on hand to boost the color and flavor of the salad, such as bell peppers, carrots, or celery. The more color variety, the more nutrients you'll consume.

Per Serving: Calories: 284; Saturated Fat: 1g; Total Fat: 10g; Protein: 14g; Total Carbs: 39g; Fiber: 13g; Sodium: 73mg

PESTO LENTILS

Serves 2

Prep time: 5 minutes

Cook time: 20 minutes

Simplicity is underrated. When you have high-quality ingredients, simple is almost always better. There's just something about the creamy pesto mixed with the tender legume here that works.

INGREDIENTS

1 cup dried brown lentils, rinsed

2 cups water

1 teaspoon salt

¼ cup Kale Walnut Pesto (page 44), Vegan Cashew Pesto (page 142), or commercially prepared pesto

4 to 8 fresh basil leaves, roughly chopped (optional)

1. In a medium pot over medium-high heat, combine the lentils, water, and salt. Cover the pot and bring the liquid to a boil. Reduce the heat to low and simmer, covered, for 20 minutes, or until the lentils are soft. Strain any excess liquid. Transfer the lentils to a large bowl.

2. Add the pesto to the lentils and toss to coat. Serve hot or cold garnished with basil (if using).

STORAGE TIP

To keep basil fresh, trim the stems and place them in a glass of water, like cut flowers. Loosely cover the leaves with a plastic bag and store on the counter. Whole basil leaves can be frozen by removing them from the stem, blanching them in boiling water for 2 seconds, and then transferring them to an ice bath. Let the blanched leaves dry completely, then wrap the leaves in parchment paper and store in a freezer-safe container.

Per Serving: Calories: 454; Saturated Fat: 2g; Total Fat: 13g; Protein: 28g; Total Carbs: 57g; Fiber: 13g; Sodium: 202mg

BLACK BEANS

In traditional Chinese medicine, black beans are considered a "warming" food that helps regulate water in the body and tonify the blood. Beans, in general, have a reputation for producing gas. Though troublesome, this gas can be attributed to starch not broken down in the intestines. This starch leads to the formation of short-chain fatty acids, which are used to feed probiotics, or the good bacteria, in your gut.

AT A GLANCE: anthocyanins, fiber, protein

HEALING POWER: Black beans are a great source of fiber, providing about 15 grams per cup. Much of this fiber is soluble fiber, which absorbs water in the gut, turning into a gel-like material and helping move things through the digestive system more easily. Black beans are a great source of vegetarian protein and combine with rice to create a complete protein source, with all essential amino acids our bodies need. The black pigment can be attributed to anthocyanins, which is the antioxidant found in foods with blue, black, and purple colors, like blueberries and red cabbage. This phytonutrient fights oxidative damage and reduces inflammation.

HEALTH BENEFITS/MEDICAL CONDITIONS: Black beans may benefit people with diabetes because the high fiber and resistant starch content can improve insulin sensitivity. The fiber and resistant starch may improve digestion and help you feel fuller longer, which may promote weight loss. The complex carbohydrates and fiber in black beans are a great source of energy for athletes. The fiber in black beans may fight inflammation and decrease the risk of inflammatory diseases, heart disease, and cancer. The resistant starch is a good source of prebiotics, which may improve gut health. The soluble fiber content may relieve constipation and can bind to cholesterol in the body, helping remove it, thereby reducing the risk of heart disease. The anthocyanins in black beans may fight cancer, especially colon cancer, and promote optimal heart health.

CONSUMPTION: 1 cup cooked black beans

BLACK BEAN SOUP

Serves 4

Prep time: 10 minutes

Cook time: 45 minutes

A simple black bean soup is a tasty way to reap the benefits from healing black beans with a ton of other health-promoting ingredients, like onion, garlic, and cumin. Soup is one of my favorite meals to make and keep in the freezer for an easy meal. Warm up with this delicious blend that will keep you full and incredibly well-nourished.

INGREDIENTS

2 tablespoons extra-virgin olive oil

1 yellow onion, chopped

2 carrots, peeled and chopped

2 celery stalks, chopped

3 garlic cloves, finely minced

2 teaspoons ground cumin

¼ teaspoon red pepper flakes

2 (15-ounce) cans no-salt-added black beans, drained and rinsed

2 cups low-sodium vegetable broth

Salt

Freshly ground black pepper

1. In a large soup pot over medium heat, heat the olive oil. Add the onion, carrots, and celery. Cook for about 10 minutes until very soft.

2. Stir in the garlic, cumin, and red pepper flakes. Cook, stirring constantly, for about 1 minute until fragrant.

3. Add the black beans and vegetable broth and bring the soup to a simmer. Reduce the heat to medium-low and cook for 25 to 30 minutes, or until the beans are tender.

4. Remove 2 cups of the soup and let cool, then blend in a high-speed blender until smooth. Return the blended soup to the pot and mix well. Taste and season with salt and pepper.

COOKING TIP

If you prefer a smoother soup, blend the whole batch. If you prefer a chunkier soup or want to cut prep time, no blending required!

Per Serving: Calories: 184; Saturated Fat: 1g; Total Fat: 7g; Protein: 9g; Total Carbs: 22g; Fiber: 8g; Sodium: 232mg

BLACK BEAN BURGERS

Serves 6

Prep time: 10 minutes

Chill time: 30 minutes

Cook time: 10 minutes

Veggie burgers are a great plant-based alternative to a traditional beef patty. Black beans provide ample fiber and oats contribute soothing and cholesterol-lowering benefits. Typical store-bought veggie burgers have a long list of ingredients, including lots of questionable preservatives. Using canned black beans is an easy way to cut cooking time, but you can cook your own black beans, if you prefer.

INGREDIENTS

2 (15-ounce) cans no-salt-added black beans, drained and rinsed

¾ cup old-fashioned rolled oats

½ cup water

2 tablespoons soy sauce

2 garlic cloves, finely minced

1 teaspoon chili powder

1 teaspoon onion powder

3 scallions, chopped finely, white and green parts

2 tablespoons avocado oil

1. In a food processor or blender, combine the black beans, oats, water, soy sauce, garlic, chili powder, and onion powder. Process until well combined.

2. Carefully remove the blade and stir in the scallions. Shape the mixture into 6 patties. Transfer to a plate, cover, and refrigerate for 30 minutes.

3. In a large skillet over medium heat, heat the avocado oil. Cook the patties, in batches if needed, for about 5 minutes per side, or until browned.

COOKING TIP

If you are pressed for time, let the patties sit at room temperature for 10 minutes instead of refrigerating them for 30 minutes.

Per Serving: Calories: 148; Saturated Fat: 1g; Total Fat: 6g; Protein: 6g; Total Carbs: 19g; Fiber: 6g; Sodium: 386mg

CHICKPEAS

These high-fiber high-protein legumes are used frequently in Middle Eastern, Mediterranean, and African cooking. They are thought to have an alkalizing effect, which can help balance high acidity levels. Aquafaba, the water in which the chickpeas have been cooked or canned, is highly nutritious and can be used similarly to egg whites in vegan cooking.

AT A GLANCE: fiber, folate, zinc

HEALING POWER: Chickpeas are a great low-calorie source of fiber and protein, as well as complex carbohydrates. The legume provides slow-releasing carbohydrates that help control blood sugar and increase satiety. Most of the fiber is insoluble fiber, which is not digested in the body, but is metabolized by bacteria in the colon to produce beneficial short-chain fatty acids, which provide fuel to intestinal cells. One cup of cooked chickpeas provides 15 grams of protein, which is more than two whole eggs. When combined with a whole grain, the chickpeas become a complete protein, providing all essential amino acids for the body's needs. Chickpeas promote fertility, as they have high levels of zinc and folate.

HEALTH BENEFITS/MEDICAL CONDITIONS: The fiber in chickpeas can help improve digestion and reduce the risk of chronic disease, including heart disease, cancer, and diabetes. Chickpeas have a low glycemic index and may improve insulin response. Consuming chickpeas may help decrease cholesterol and other markers related to heart disease and may promote weight loss, as they are low in calories but high in protein and fiber. They are a good vegetarian source of protein. Folate and zinc may improve male-factor fertility and improve sperm concentration in men.

CONSUMPTION: 1 cup cooked chickpeas

BAKED GREEN FALAFEL BITES

Serves 3
Prep time: 10 minutes
Cook time: 30 minutes

These baked falafels have all the powerful protein and filling fiber of chickpeas, without the added oil typically used in a deep-fried preparation. Cilantro and parsley do double duty, boosting flavor and helping fight inflammation. These bites can be enjoyed on their own as a plant-based snack or used as the centerpiece of a main dish.

INGREDIENTS

2 (15-ounce) cans no-salt-added chickpeas, drained and rinsed

½ red onion, quartered

2 garlic cloves, minced

½ cup fresh parsley

½ cup fresh cilantro

¼ cup extra-virgin olive oil

1 teaspoon red pepper flakes

1 teaspoon sea salt

½ teaspoon freshly ground black pepper

½ teaspoon ground cumin

1. Preheat the oven to 375°F. Line a large rimmed sheet pan with parchment paper or a silicone baking mat. Set aside.

2. In a food processor, combine the chickpeas, red onion, garlic, parsley, cilantro, olive oil, red pepper flakes, salt, pepper, and cumin. Process until smooth.

3. Using an ice cream scoop, a spoon, or your hands, make 6 small patties, about 2 inches in diameter, and place them on the prepared sheet pan.

4. Bake for 30 minutes, or until the falafels ae golden on top and cooked through. Let cool.

STORAGE TIP

Refrigerate in an airtight container for up to 4 days, or freeze for 2 to 3 months.

Per Serving: Calories: 432; Saturated Fat: 3g; Total Fat: 21g; Protein: 15g; Total Carbs: 49g; Fiber: 14g; Sodium: 544mg

ROASTED CHICKPEAS

Serves 10

Prep time: 10 minutes
Cook time: 45 minutes

Roasted chickpeas are a great protein- and fiber-filled snack and are a delicious, crunchy salad topper. Swap these for your typical croutons to improve your salad game. Change the spices for savory or sweet chickpeas.

INGREDIENTS

2 (15-ounce) cans no-salt-added chickpeas, drained and rinsed

2 tablespoons extra-virgin olive oil

1 teaspoon sea salt

1. Preheat the oven to 400°F.

2. Spread the chickpeas on a clean dishtowel and dry them well. Transfer the chickpeas to a baking sheet, drizzle with olive oil, and sprinkle with salt. Mix well, tossing to coat each chickpea.

3. Bake for 45 minutes, or until golden and crispy.

4. Store the roasted chickpeas in an airtight container at room temperature for up to 1 week (if they last that long)!

VARIATION TIP

Add different spices to change the flavor profile, such as garlic, onion, cumin, cinnamon, or cayenne.

Per Serving: Calories: 105; Saturated Fat: 1g; Total Fat: 4g; Protein: 4g; Total Carbs: 14g; Fiber: 4g; Sodium: 191mg

ALMONDS

Almonds are technically the seeds of a fruit that grows on the almond tree, and are related to peaches, cherries, and apricots. They are thought to have originated in Asia, and then traveled along the Silk Road to the Mediterranean. In ancient Rome, newlyweds were showered with almonds to promote fertility for the new couple. Almonds are used in Ayurvedic medicine to improve the health of the nervous system and the brain. Almond oil is used topically in Ayurvedic and traditional Chinese medicine to treat psoriasis and eczema.

AT A GLANCE: calcium, flavonoids, magnesium, monounsaturated fat, vitamin E

HEALING POWER: Almonds are an incredibly healing food with regard to heart health because of their antioxidants and protein content. Almonds are also a great source of monounsaturated fats, which promote satiety and improve the absorption of fat-soluble vitamins. Almonds can help lower cholesterol, specifically LDL (the "bad") cholesterol. Almonds are rich in vitamin E, an antioxidant that helps protect cells from oxidative damage. There are also antioxidants, called flavonoids, in the skin of almonds, which work in tandem with vitamin E to fight free radicals and reduce inflammation. The magnesium in almonds benefits almost every bodily process and enhances the absorption of calcium, which can help promote strong bones.

HEALTH BENEFITS/MEDICAL CONDITIONS: When consumed in small amounts, almonds may help promote weight loss. Celebrated as a heart-healthy nut, almonds can help improve blood pressure and lower LDL cholesterol. Consuming almonds provides antioxidants, which can reduce inflammation in the body and prevent chronic diseases such as cancer. The healthy fats, fiber, and magnesium in almonds may help promote blood sugar control, helping people with diabetes. Almonds are a good source of calcium for those who are lactose intolerant or vegan. Almond oil can be used topically to help soothe skin and reduce scarring.

CONSUMPTION: 1 ounce, ¼ cup, or about 23 almonds

HOMEMADE ROASTED MAPLE
ALMOND BUTTER

Makes about 1 ½ cups

Prep time: 5 minutes

Cook time: 30 minutes

In my opinion, there's nothing better than almond butter. Well, maybe maple almond butter! Justin's Maple Almond Butter packets are one of my favorite on-the-go snacks to eat with fresh fruit and I frequently squeeze it into a cup of oatmeal for a quick breakfast. Making your own almond butter at home is easy! Almonds are great for blood sugar control, and by making your own nut butter, you control how much (or how little) sweetener you include.

INGREDIENTS

2 cups raw almonds

¼ cup maple syrup

1 teaspoon vanilla extract

½ teaspoon salt

1. Preheat the oven to 300°F. Line a baking sheet with parchment paper or a silicone baking mat.

2. In a medium bowl, stir together the almonds, maple syrup, vanilla, and salt. Spread the almonds into a single layer on the prepared baking sheet.

3. Bake for 30 minutes, stirring halfway through the baking time. Let cool for 10 minutes.

4. Transfer the almonds to a food processor or high-speed blender. Process for about 5 minutes, or until you have achieved the desired consistency, stopping to scrape down the sides, as needed.

INGREDIENT TIP

Go nuts with bulk bins! Purchasing organic raw nuts in bulk can be a less expensive way to purchase the quantity of nuts you need for a specific recipe. To preserve the quality of the nuts, keep them refrigerated.

Per Serving (1 tablespoon): Calories: 77; Saturated Fat: 9g; Total Fat: 9g; Protein: 3g; Total Carbs: 5g; Fiber: 2g; Sodium: 51mg

SIMPLE ALMOND TRAIL MIX

Makes about 3 ½ cups

Prep time: 5 minutes

Making your own trail mix is a great way to have a healthy snack on hand at all times. This trail mix is also a delicious topper for smoothies, salads, and parfaits. You can include whatever nuts and seeds you like, but steer clear of sweetened dried fruits to avoid excess sugar in your diet. Brazil nuts can help provide your daily needs of selenium, an essential mineral for thyroid and immune function.

INGREDIENTS

1 cup raw almonds

1 cup raw Brazil nuts

½ cup raw cashews

½ cup pumpkin seeds

½ cup sunflower seeds

½ teaspoon ground cinnamon

¼ teaspoon sea salt

Pinch ground nutmeg

In a large bowl, combine the almonds, Brazil nuts, cashews, pumpkin seeds, sunflower seeds, cinnamon, salt, and nutmeg. Mix well. Store in a large jar, sealed well, at room temperature, or divide into individual servings and store in resealable bags.

STORAGE TIP

Consider purchasing a reusable snack bag, such as the silicone Stasher, for a more environmentally friendly alternative to plastic.

Per Serving (½ cup): Calories: 374; Saturated Fat: 6g; Total Fat: 33g; Protein: 12g; Total Carbs: 12g; Fiber: 5g; Sodium: 70mg

PEAS

Peas have been in the spotlight recently with the emergence of many pea-based products, like pea protein powder, but peas have been around for centuries. A bag of frozen peas may be a simple cooling therapy to a bruise, but there is a lot of nutrition packed into those bright green globes. In the Ayurvedic tradition, peas are thought to be beneficial to the colon and are used medicinally to promote digestion. Like other bright green vegetables, peas pack an antioxidant punch and can be used to fight inflammation.

AT A GLANCE: chlorophyll, fiber, iron, protein, vitamin C

HEALING POWER: According to the USDA, 1 cup of peas provides about 8.5 grams of protein. That's more than one whole egg! This protein comes along with iron, which helps improve energy and ensures your tissues and muscles get enough oxygen. Peas also are a great digestive aid and can be used for their soothing and laxative powers. The dietary fiber in peas helps bulk stool and move it through the digestive tract. Peas have great anti-oxidant powers due to their vitamin C, but also chlorophyll, the green pigment that gives peas their color. Chlorophyll helps detoxify the liver, support the immune system, and prevent cancer.

HEALTH BENEFITS/MEDICAL CONDITIONS: Peas are high in fiber, which may help prevent digestive issues and reduce the risk of heart disease. Dietary fiber helps reduce and eliminate cholesterol, lowering the risk of heart disease and stroke. The protein and fiber in peas may help with weight management, as they can help promote satiety and make you feel fuller longer. The vitamin C content in peas may help prevent colds and reduce the risk of cancer. The chlorophyll in peas may boost the immune system. The iron in peas may help prevent anemia, and is helpful for pregnant and lactating women.

CONSUMPTION: 1 cup peas

PEA AND LETTUCE SOUP

Serves 4
Prep time: 15 minutes
Cook time: 15 minutes

Yes, peas! Soup is a great way to reap the benefits of vegetables and legumes. This creamy green soup tastes incredibly indulgent and is surprisingly filling as a result of its high fiber content. Shallots and fennel create depth of flavor and help the body detoxify.

INGREDIENTS

2 tablespoons extra-virgin olive oil

1 fennel bulb, cored and chopped

2 small shallots, chopped

1 Bibb lettuce head, roughly chopped

2 cups low-sodium vegetable broth

1 (10-ounce) package frozen peas

½ cup water

1 teaspoon sea salt

1 teaspoon freshly ground black pepper

½ cup pumpkin seeds

1. In a large saucepan over medium heat, heat the olive oil. Add the fennel and shallots. Cook for about 5 minutes until tender, stirring periodically.

2. Add the lettuce and cook for about 1 minute, mixing constantly, until wilted.

3. Stir in the vegetable broth, peas, water, salt, and pepper. Bring the soup to a boil, cover the pan, and reduce the heat to low. Simmer for 5 minutes until the peas are tender. Let the soup cool slightly.

4. Working in batches, carefully transfer the soup to a blender and process until smooth. Top each serving with 2 tablespoons of pumpkin seeds.

COOKING TIP

For easy pre-prepped meals, double the recipe and freeze half! This soup is delicious served with a side salad or a slice of sourdough bread.

Per Serving: Calories: 250; Saturated Fat: 15g; Total Fat: 3g; Protein: 10g; Total Carbs: 22g; Fiber: 7g; Sodium: 563mg

PEA HUMMUS

Makes about 2 cups
Prep time: 5 minutes
Cook time: 5 minutes

You've likely seen varieties of chickpea hummus and black bean hummus—but pea hummus? It's a game changer! Green peas are low in calories, but high in protein and fiber. Serve with toasted whole-wheat pita bread or carrots and celery.

INGREDIENTS

2 cups frozen green peas, thawed

¼ cup extra-virgin olive oil

2 tablespoons tahini

Juice of ½ lemon

1 garlic clove, roughly chopped

½ teaspoon salt

1. Bring a small pot of water to a boil over high heat. Add the peas and cook for about 2 minutes until tender. Drain. Transfer the peas to a food processor.

2. Add the olive oil, tahini, lemon juice, garlic, and salt. Blend for about 1 minute, or until smooth. Season as desired.

VARIATION TIP

For a flavor boost, add ¼ teaspoon ground cumin to the blend.

Per Serving (2 tablespoons): Calories: 53; Saturated Fat: 1g; Total Fat: 4g; Protein: 1g; Total Carbs: 3g; Fiber: 1g; Sodium: 77mg

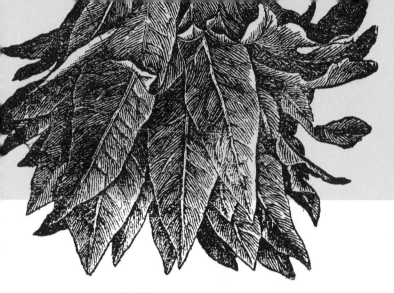

CORN BEYOND THE COB

Corn is an incredibly versatile legume, and although much of the corn produced in the United States is used for human and animal feed, there are many alternative uses. You know you can eat it on the cob, as popcorn, or in a salad, but did you know all the ways this food staple is used aside from food consumption? Corn is used as ethanol in the oil and gas industry. It's also used to make an environmentally friendly plastic. Cornstarch, a common baking ingredient, is used in cosmetics, such as deodorant, and is found in medications as a binder or in the coating. Glue and other adhesives used in things like wallpaper, and even paint, typically contain cornmeal or cornstarch. Although you can still make a corncob pipe for a snowman, today corncobs are also used to make various absorbents for oil and waste materials.

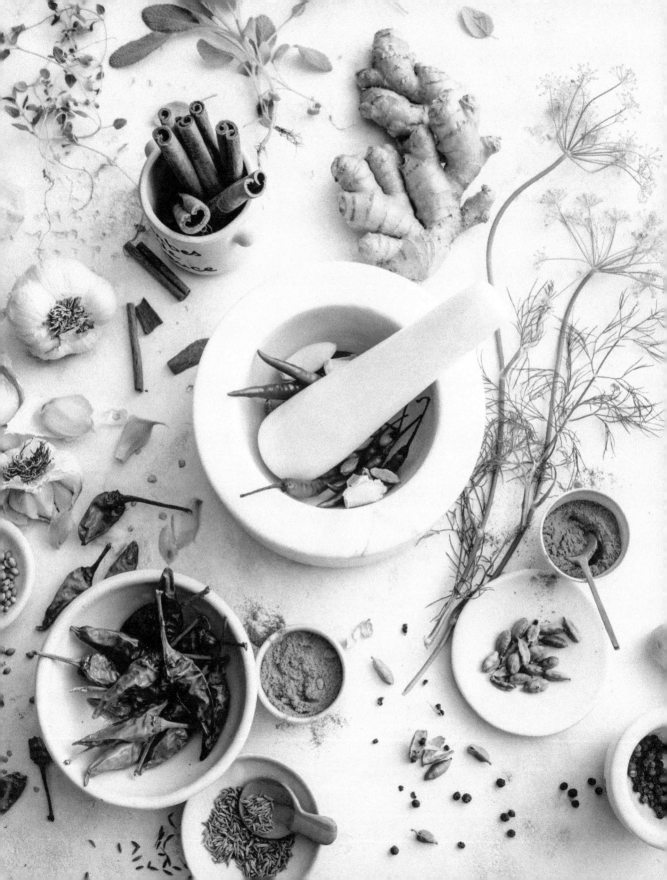

6

Herbs and Spices

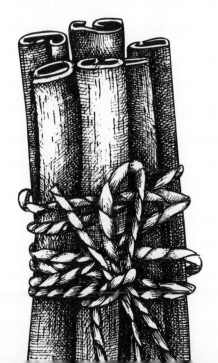

If you're looking to heal a stomachache or reduce inflammation, don't forget to look in your spice cabinet for help. Early cultures used herbs and spices to heal common ailments, and even today, plants are a key component of many pharmaceutical drugs. Despite the advances in conventional medicine, there is a resurgence of focus on herbal remedies, and many people are looking beyond the medicine cabinet for complementary remedies. In this chapter, I profile 10 healing herbs and spices you can integrate into your diet to heal various concerns.

MINT

Peppermint has long been used to relieve gas and bloating. Although a renowned digestive aid, especially when brewed in tea, mint is also used to treat nausea. Many pregnant women can avoid sensitivity to smell by chewing mint-flavored gum or smelling something minty. Some people think that chewing peppermint leaves can relieve a toothache. Note that although mint is a powerful digestive aid, it can also be a trigger for those with acid reflux, making digestive issues worse for them.

AT A GLANCE: luteolin, menthol, menthoside

HEALING POWER: Peppermint works therapeutically as a digestive aid to relieve pain and muscle spasm. Peppermint is shown to relax the gastrointestinal tissue, which may help relieve digestive distress and reduce nausea, cramps, and gas. Menthol, a powerful volatile oil found in peppermint's leaves, is known for its cooling capacities, both internally and externally. Peppermint also contains flavonoids such as luteolin and menthoside, which work as antioxidants in the body and help reduce inflammation. Peppermint can relieve and reduce sensitivity to pain.

HEALTH BENEFITS/MEDICAL CONDITIONS: The menthol in peppermint may help treat digestive issues such as cramps, nausea, gas, and bloating. It helps relieve a spastic colon, which is soothing for diarrhea and constipation, as well as other symptoms of inflammatory bowel diseases and irritable bowel syndrome. Peppermint may help provide relief from menstrual cramps, as well as general pain, especially for headaches and migraines when the essential oil is applied topically. Menthol found in peppermint is used frequently in chest rubs for respiratory infections. Peppermint is a great way to freshen breath and may relieve fatigue.

CONSUMPTION: 1 teaspoon dried, or 2 teaspoons fresh, per 1 cup of water up to 3 times per day

FRESH MINT TEA

Serves 2

Prep time: 5 minutes

Cook time: 5 minutes

This simple tea is incredibly refreshing and naturally caffeine free. Technically, it is classified as a tisane, as it is made from fresh leaves other than *Camellia sinensis* (the plant traditional tea comes from; see page 174). Mint is great for easing stomach woes, improving sleep, and relieving clogged sinuses.

INGREDIENTS

2 cups water

10 fresh peppermint leaves

1 to 2 teaspoons honey (optional)

2 lemon slices

1. In a small saucepan over high heat, bring the water to a boil. Remove from the heat, add the mint leaves, and steep for 5 minutes.

2. Strain out the leaves, stir in the honey (if using), and serve with lemon slices.

VARIATION TIP

Use a different citrus fruit, such as orange or grapefruit, to flavor the herbal tea. Other varieties of mint can also be used, such as spearmint.

Per Serving: Calories: 4; Saturated Fat: 0g; Total Fat: 0g; Protein: 0g; Total Carbs: 1g; Fiber: 0g; Sodium: 0mg

MINT CHOCOLATE CHIP SMOOTHIE

Serves 1

Prep time: 5 minutes

This blend tastes too good to be healthy, but it is! It's packed with fiber, antioxidants, and iron. It's great for breakfast but can also be enjoyed in place of an after-dinner dessert (you may want to share it . . . or not) because the magnesium in the cacao nibs helps promote relaxation and sleep.

INGREDIENTS

1 cup unsweetened plain almond milk

1 cup fresh baby spinach

1 banana, peeled and frozen

10 fresh mint leaves

1 tablespoon cacao nibs, plus extra for topping (optional)

½ teaspoon vanilla extract

3 or 4 ice cubes

In a high-speed blender, combine the almond milk, spinach, banana, mint, cacao nibs, vanilla, and ice. Blend on high speed until smooth. Top with a sprinkle, about 1 teaspoon, of cacao nibs (if using) for extra crunch.

COOKING TIP

If you didn't have time to freeze the banana, use a fresh ripe banana and add an extra ice cube or two to achieve your desired consistency.

SUBSTITUTION TIP

If you can't find cacao nibs, substitute 1 tablespoon cacao powder.

Per Serving: Calories: 207; Saturated Fat: 0g; Total Fat: 7g; Protein: 5g; Total Carbs: 32g; Fiber: 7g; Sodium: 389mg

BASIL

There are many varieties of this herb, including sweet basil, Thai basil, and holy basil. Sweet basil is used mostly for cooking (and we will focus on this varietal), whereas holy basil, also called tulsi, is used in various supplements. In Roman times, sweet basil was used to counteract poisoning, relieve gas, and promote lactation in breastfeeding mothers. Sweet basil is used widely in Ayurvedic medicine as a digestive aid. Topically, the leaves can be used as an insect repellent.

AT A GLANCE: eugenol, magnesium, vitamin K

HEALING POWER: Basil can be used to treat gas, stomach cramps, and indigestion. These stomach-quelling properties of basil may be attributed to eugenol, a phenolic compound with incredible anti-inflammatory and pain-relieving capabilities. Eugenol is also a powerful antioxidant that helps fight free radicals in the body. Magnesium in basil may also promote a calming effect on the nervous system. Basil contains antibacterial properties, which can be used to inhibit infection.

HEALTH BENEFITS/MEDICAL CONDITIONS: The volatile oils in basil, like eugenol, may reduce inflammation and the incidence of inflammatory diseases such as arthritis and heart disease. The anti-inflammatory constituents in basil may reduce inflammation in the digestive tract and relieve stomach pain and indigestion. The magnesium in basil may reduce irritability, depression, and anxiety. Magnesium also helps promote cardiovascular health by improving blood flow and reducing the risk of irregular heart contractions. Eugenol in basil acts as an antioxidant and can help prevent cancer. The antibacterial properties of basil may boost the immune system and protect against infections.

CONSUMPTION: 2 tablespoons fresh basil, or 1½ teaspoons dried

VEGAN CASHEW PESTO

Serves 6

Prep time: 5 minutes

Traditional pesto recipes call for cheese, but this recipe does not, making it dairy-free and vegan. The miso adds salty, savory flavor and provides beneficial bacteria for a healthy gut. This pesto is delicious with any steamed vegetable, grain, or pasta. I recommend making pesto zucchini noodles or Pesto Lentils (page 121).

INGREDIENTS

2 cups fresh basil leaves

½ cup raw unsalted cashews

Juice of ½ lemon

1 tablespoon light miso paste

2 garlic cloves, peeled

¼ teaspoon salt

¼ cup extra-virgin olive oil, plus more
  as needed

In a food processor, combine the basil, cashews, lemon juice, miso, garlic, and salt. With the processor running, gradually stream in the olive oil and process until well combined.

VARIATION TIP

You can toast the nuts in a skillet over medium heat for 2 minutes if you would like more flavor. Let them cool before combining.

Per Serving: Calories: 138; Saturated Fat: 2g; Total Fat: 13g; Protein: 2g; Total Carbs: 4g; Fiber: 1g; Sodium: 204mg

GARLIC

The ancient Romans and Greeks believed garlic had magical powers and, to some extent, it does! Garlic is a powerful treatment for a host of ailments ranging from colds to asthma and arthritis. The Greeks used garlic as a "performance-enhancing drug" and gave it to athletes who competed in the first Olympics. In traditional Chinese medicine, garlic is used to improve respiration and digestion. In ancient India, garlic was used as a treatment for fatigue and parasites. Prior to the invention of antibiotics, garlic was used as a treatment for almost every infection.

AT A GLANCE: allicin, vitamins C and E

HEALING POWER: Garlic is a natural antibiotic, expectorant, and decongestant. Although researchers are still studying the precise mechanism of garlic's medicinal effects, allicin is touted as the powerful antiseptic constituent. Found in the volatile oil of garlic, allicin is produced when garlic is chopped or crushed. This compound has incredible anti-inflammatory and antioxidant benefits. The antioxidant benefits are amplified by garlic's vitamins C and E.

HEALTH BENEFITS/MEDICAL CONDITIONS: Consuming garlic may help improve heart health by preventing atherosclerosis, reducing cholesterol and triglyceride levels, and reducing blood pressure. As a result of lowered cholesterol and blood pressure, garlic can help prevent circulatory problems and strokes. Garlic may help prevent cold and flu, as well as earaches and coughs. The antimicrobial properties of garlic may help fight bacterial infections, including E. coli and salmonella. Sulfuric compounds in garlic may help reduce the risk of various cancers. Allicin found in garlic also has antifungal properties and can be used internally and externally to treat fungal skin conditions, like athlete's foot.

CONSUMPTION: 2 or 3 cloves

ROASTED GARLIC DRESSING

Makes about 1 cup

Prep time: 5 minutes

Cook time: 45 minutes

There's nothing more delicious than roasted garlic right out of the oven. The smell alone can make you swoon, but the cold-fighting compounds and medicinal qualities of garlic are definitely something to cheer. This versatile dressing can be used on salads, vegetables, or grains or as a dip for sourdough bread.

INGREDIENTS

2 large garlic heads

⅓ cup plus 2 tablespoons extra-virgin olive oil, divided

¼ cup red wine vinegar

2 tablespoons freshly squeezed lemon juice

Salt

Freshly ground black pepper

1. Preheat the oven to 400°F.

2. Cut off the tips of the stem end of the garlic heads to expose the cloves, keeping the head intact. Place the garlic on a piece of aluminum foil. Drizzle the cloves with olive oil, about 1 tablespoon per head, and tightly wrap the heads in the foil.

3. Bake for 45 minutes. Unwrap and let cool.

4. Separate the roasted garlic pulp from their skins by squeezing the pulp from the skin. Discard the skins.

5. In a high-speed blender, combine the garlic pulp with the remaining ⅓ cup of olive oil, the vinegar, and lemon juice. Season with salt and pepper. Blend until smooth.

STORAGE TIP

Freeze roasted garlic cloves for future use in sauces or dressings. Mash the roasted garlic cloves, then place them in an empty ice cube tray and cover. Freeze, then transfer the cubes to an airtight bag or container.

Per Serving (2 tablespoons): Calories: 134; Saturated Fat: 2g; Total Fat: 14g; Protein: 1g; Total Carbs: 3g; Fiber: 0g; Sodium: 22mg

GARLIC-GINGER ROASTED BROCCOLI

Serves 4

Prep time: 10 minutes

Cook time: 20 minutes

Did you ever wonder why so many recipes call for garlic that is minced, crushed, or chopped? A special compound, allicin, is produced during these preparations. The allicin in garlic may reduce inflammation and have an antibacterial effect. Although garlic is a bit harsh to eat alone, this winning combination of ginger, broccoli, and garlic is unbeatable.

INGREDIENTS

2 broccoli heads (about 1 pound)

2 tablespoons extra-virgin olive oil

2 tablespoons grated peeled fresh ginger

2 tablespoons finely minced garlic

Salt

Freshly ground black pepper

1. Preheat the oven to 425°F. Line a baking sheet with parchment paper.

2. Cut the broccoli into florets. Peel the stalks and cut them into ½-inch chunks. Transfer to a large bowl.

3. Add the olive oil, ginger, and garlic. Season with salt and pepper. Toss to coat and combine. Transfer the mixture to the prepared baking sheet and spread it into an even layer.

4. Roast for 15 to 20 minutes, or until the broccoli is browned.

COOKING TIP

Use frozen broccoli if you prefer. No need to thaw, just roast for 20 minutes, flip, then roast for 5 to 10 minutes more, or until the broccoli is browned.

Per Serving: Calories: 107; Saturated Fat: 1g; Total Fat: 7g; Protein: 4g; Total Carbs: 9g; Fiber: 3g; Sodium: 77mg

PARSLEY

Parsley has been used throughout history as a natural diuretic, helping the body eliminate excess fluid. The ancient Romans and Greeks used parsley for this reason, but also as a digestive tonic and menstrual stimulant. Normally used as a garnish, parsley is actually an incredibly nutritious salad herb native to the Mediterranean region that can be used medicinally to treat a host of ailments.

AT A GLANCE: apiole, folic acid, myristicin, vitamin C

HEALING POWER: The diuretic properties of parsley can be attributed to the myristicin and apiole found in parsley's volatile oil. These components increase the flow of urine, which removes excess fluid from the body and can prevent urinary tract infections. Apiole is also thought to be an emmenagogue, or stimulator of menstruation. Parsley also contains flavonoids, including apigenin, which have antioxidant and anti-inflammatory effects in the body and, along with parsley's vitamin C content, help reverse free radical damage. The folic acid in parsley helps reduce the amount of blood vessel–damaging homocysteine found in the body.

HEALTH BENEFITS/MEDICAL CONDITIONS: The diuretic effects of parsley may reduce water retention and bloating. This decrease in bloating may be helpful for those who struggle with premenstrual syndrome. The antioxidant and anti-inflammatory flavonoids in parsley help reduce the risk of cancer, reduce systemic inflammation, and promote immune function. Reduced inflammation may benefit people with arthritis, allergies, autoimmune disorders, and other chronic inflammatory diseases. Parsley may help those with an irregular period. For those who are pregnant, the folate content in parsley may help protect against birth defects. Parsley is also a natural breath freshener.

CONSUMPTION: ½ cup chopped

CHIMICHURRI

Makes about 1 cup

Prep time: 5 minutes, plus 20 minutes for marinating

Chimichurri adds loads of nutrition and flavor to any dish. No matter the season, you can choose any assortment of vegetables, roast them, and then top them with chimichurri for a delicious flavor boost. The versatile sauce is also delicious when mixed with cooked whole grains or legume pasta for an easy weeknight meal.

INGREDIENTS

½ cup extra-virgin olive oil

¼ cup chopped fresh parsley

3 tablespoons red wine vinegar

4 garlic cloves, peeled

2 tablespoons dried oregano

1 tablespoon red pepper flakes

1 teaspoon sea salt

In a food processor, combine the olive oil, parsley, vinegar, garlic, oregano, red pepper flakes, and salt. Process until smooth. Let sit, covered, for at least 20 minutes before serving.

STORAGE TIP

Refrigerate in an airtight container for 1 week. To freeze chimichurri, pour the sauce into an ice cube tray, freeze, then transfer the cubes to an airtight container in the freezer and use within 3 months.

Per Serving (2 tablespoons): Calories: 118; Saturated Fat: 2g; Total Fat: 13g; Protein: 0g; Total Carbs: 2g; Fiber: 1g; Sodium: 236mg

CAULIFLOWER WITH LEMON, CAPERS, AND PARSLEY

Serves 4

Prep time: 10 minutes

Cook time: 30 minutes

Bright green parsley boosts the nutrition, flavor, and color of this zesty cauliflower dish. Many times this common herb is regarded simply as a garnish, with parsley's nutrient power often overlooked. Not here! The flavors meld to create an antioxidant-rich, detoxifying side with parsley as a star.

INGREDIENTS

1 cauliflower head, cut into florets

3 tablespoons extra-virgin olive oil

Salt

Freshly ground black pepper

½ cup chopped fresh parsley

Juice of ½ lemon

1 tablespoon grated lemon zest

1 tablespoon capers

1. Preheat the oven to 425°F.

2. In a large bowl, toss together the cauliflower and olive oil to coat. Season with salt and pepper and transfer to a baking sheet.

3. Roast the cauliflower for 30 minutes until lightly browned and softened.

4. Transfer the cauliflower to a serving bowl and toss with the parsley, lemon juice, lemon zest, and capers.

INGREDIENT TIP

Look for cauliflower with tightly packed heads and no brown spots. If storing the cauliflower a plastic bag in the refrigerator, keep the bag open to prevent moisture from gathering and accelerating spoilage.

Per Serving: Calories: 111; Saturated Fat: 2g; Total Fat: 11g; Protein: 2g; Total Carbs: 4g; Fiber: 2g; Sodium: 128mg

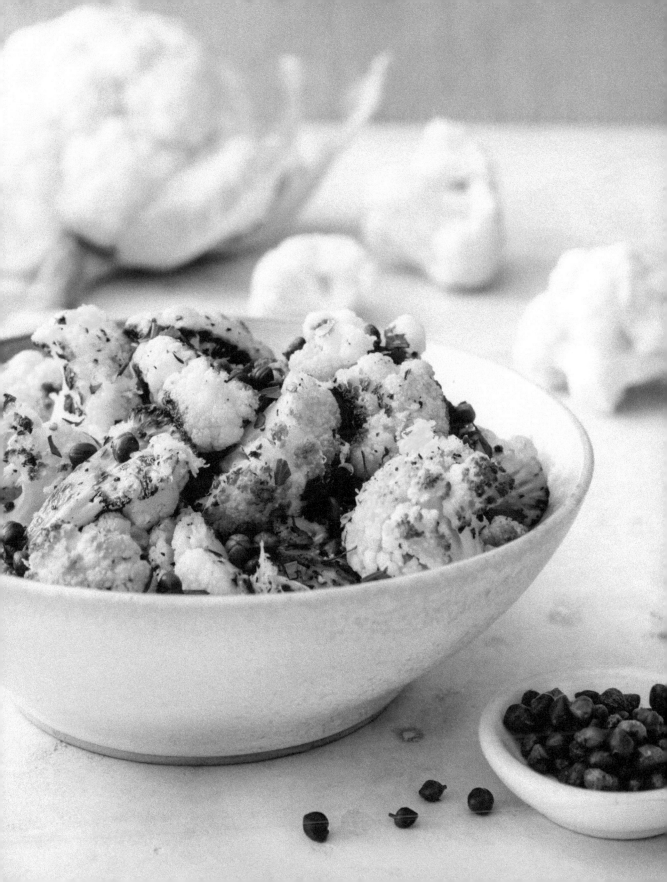

LAVENDER

Lavender-scented candles and soaps help create a relaxing home environment. But, did you know lavender has healing properties, too? In the Middle Ages, lavender was used as a medicine for headaches and joint pain. The flowers are now used widely in essential oils, massage oils, and teas for anxiety relief. Culinary lavender is used in baking and to create infused cooking oils and relaxation-promoting teas.

AT A GLANCE: linalool, linalyl acetate, flavonoids

HEALING POWER: Lavender flowers have antiseptic and anti-inflammatory powers. Two phytochemicals found in the essential oil of the flowers, linalyl acetate and linalool, are anti-inflammatory and can help relieve pain and fight inflammation. These phytochemicals can also reduce swelling related to insect bites and burns. When used as a calming remedy for digestive problems, lavender helps relieve indigestion and relax the muscles in the gastrointestinal tract. Lavender has sedative properties that help calm the nervous system, reduce feelings of anxiety, and promote a relaxed mood.

HEALTH BENEFITS/MEDICAL CONDITIONS: The anti-inflammatory phytochemicals in lavender may provide relief of indigestion, bloating, and gas. When lavender essential oil is used topically, lavender's properties may reduce pain. Lavender can be used to treat insect bites or relieve a headache. It is also helpful when used with massage to promote the relaxation of stiff, aching muscles and joints. Lavender calms the nervous system and can help relieve insomnia, anxiety, and depression. It may improve sleep and can be used topically to soothe skin, so it may be good to use if you have acne or a blemish.

CONSUMPTION: ½ to 1 teaspoon

LAVENDER-INFUSED COCONUT OIL FREEZER BARK

Serves 8

Prep time: 5 minutes

Cook time: 1 hour, plus 2 hours freeze time

Coconut oil freezer bark is the cure for any chocolate craving. Infusing the coconut oil with lavender adds another flavor dimension. Coconut oil melts at room temperature, so store this treat in the freezer to prevent melting.

INGREDIENTS

½ cup coconut oil

2 tablespoons dried food-grade lavender

½ cup cacao powder

¼ cup maple syrup, at room temperature

Sea salt

COOKING TIP

If you want to infuse coconut oil naturally, combine the dried food-grade lavender and coconut oil in a Mason jar and let it sit for 20 to 30 days. When you want to use it, heat the jar to melt the oil, then strain the lavender out of the oil before using.

1. In a Mason jar, combine the coconut oil and lavender. Place the Mason jar's lid in a small saucepan and set the jar on top of the lid. Fill the saucepan halfway with water.

2. Bring the water to a boil. Reduce the heat to low and simmer for 1 hour.

3. Remove the Mason jar from the water. Strain the hot oil through a fine-mesh sieve set over a bowl. Discard the lavender.

4. Line a small loaf pan with parchment paper and set aside.

5. In a medium bowl, stir together the infused coconut oil, cacao powder, and maple syrup. Using a silicone spatula, scrape down the sides of the bowl and stir until combined. Pour the coconut-cacao mixture into the prepared loaf pan, distributing it evenly.

6. Sprinkle salt on top. Cover the pan and place it in the freezer for at least 2 hours. When fully frozen, cut or break the bark into pieces.

Per Serving: Calories: 193; Saturated Fat: 14g; Total Fat: 18g; Protein: 4g; Total Carbs: 17g; Fiber: 6g; Sodium: 1mg

LAVENDER AND MINT ICED TEA

Serves 4
Prep time: 10 minutes
Cook time: 10 minutes

There's nothing more refreshing than an ice-cold mint tea. The lavender in this version creates an aromatic, instantly relaxing sensation that turns your typical tea into a luxurious experience. Sip this soothing beverage for a sense of calm and coolness.

INGREDIENTS

1 cup fresh mint leaves

5 tablespoons dried food-grade lavender

4 cups water

Ice

1. In a medium saucepan, combine the mint leaves, lavender, and water. Place the pan over high heat and bring to a boil. Reduce the heat to maintain a simmer and cook for 10 minutes.

2. Using a fine-mesh sieve set over a pitcher or bowl, strain the lavender and mint from the tea. Let cool and serve the tea over ice.

STORAGE TIP

Use leftover iced tea to make lavender-mint ice cubes. Freeze the tea in ice cube trays, then transfer the cubes an airtight container in the freezer. The flavored ice cubes are a great way to spice up a regular glass of filtered water.

Per Serving: Calories: 2; Saturated Fat: 0g; Total Fat: 0g; Protein: 0g; Total Carbs: 0g; Fiber: 0g; Sodium: 0mg

CINNAMON

You may not think that the simple sprinkle of this sweet spice does much, but cinnamon is actually one of the most medicinal and healing spices in the world. In traditional Chinese medicine, cinnamon is a warming spice used to improve circulation, as well as cold and flu symptoms. Note that there are different types of cinnamon available—when possible, select the Ceylon variety.

AT A GLANCE: cinnamaldehyde, mucilage, procyanidins

HEALING POWER: True to its roots in Chinese tradition, cinnamon does have a warming, stimulating effect on circulation. It is a digestive aid that helps promote the digestion of fat and can be used as a calming tonic for indigestion. Cinnamon is widely celebrated for its antidiabetic powers. It helps stabilize blood sugar and may improve cells' insulin response and prevent insulin resistance. Cinnamon is also recognized for its ability to lower cholesterol. The procyanidins in cinnamon have antioxidant powers that help fight free radicals and reduce inflammation throughout the body. Cinnamaldehyde works as an antibacterial and antifungal agent, protecting against infection. This phytochemical also makes cinnamon a great way to freshen your breath.

HEALTH BENEFITS/MEDICAL CONDITIONS: The antioxidant content in cinnamon may reduce inflammation in the body and help protect against inflammatory diseases such as arthritis, cancer, and heart disease. Cinnamon may help reduce cholesterol and blood pressure, which can lower the risk of heart disease. Cinnamon may improve insulin sensitivity, helping promote blood glucose control, which is beneficial for those with diabetes and polycystic ovary syndrome. The blood glucose–controlling properties of cinnamon may promote weight loss and prevent metabolic disease. Cinnamon can be a remedy for nausea and indigestion, as it stimulates digestion and improves circulation.

CONSUMPTION: 1 to 2 teaspoons, ground

CINNAMON SPICE MAPLE WALNUTS

Makes 2 cups
Prep time: 5 minutes
Cook time: 15 minutes

If you're looking for a smart holiday or housewarming gift, look no further. Walnuts work wonders for the brain with their high content of plant-based omega-3s (they even *look* like mini brains)! Sweeten up this nutritious nut with some maple syrup and seasonal spices including cinnamon, cardamom, and nutmeg.

INGREDIENTS

2 tablespoons maple syrup

2 tablespoons coconut sugar

1 tablespoon coconut oil, melted

2 cups raw walnut halves

1½ teaspoons ground cinnamon

½ teaspoon ground nutmeg

½ teaspoon ground cardamom

Pinch sea salt

1. Preheat the oven to 375°F. Line a rimmed sheet pan with parchment paper.

2. In a bowl, stir together the maple syrup, coconut sugar, and coconut oil until well mixed. Add the walnuts, cinnamon, nutmeg, and cardamom. Toss well to combine.

3. Transfer the nuts to the prepared sheet pan and spread them into a single layer. Sprinkle with salt.

4. Bake for 15 minutes until the walnuts are lightly browned and fragrant.

INGREDIENT TIP

Store shelled or unshelled nuts in the refrigerator or freezer to prevent spoilage.

Per Serving (¼ cup): Calories: 241; Saturated Fat: 4g; Total Fat: 22g; Protein: 5g; Total Carbs: 11g; Fiber: 2g; Sodium: 43mg

TAHINI DATE CINNAMON SMOOTHIE

Serves 1

Prep time: 5 minutes

Tahini, a paste made from sesame seeds, is the base of this creamy cinnamon smoothie. Tahini is a great source of satiating healthy fats and, surprisingly, calcium. The calcium content of this smoothie makes it a great option for pregnant women or anyone looking to promote bone health.

INGREDIENTS

1 cup unsweetened plain almond milk

1 banana, peeled and frozen

¼ cup tahini

1 pitted Medjool date

1 tablespoon cacao powder

2 teaspoons ground cinnamon

In a high-speed blender, combine the almond milk, banana, tahini, date, cacao powder, and cinnamon. Blend on high speed until smooth.

INGREDIENT TIP

You can use other date varieties. If the date is not soft, soak it in hot water for 1 to 2 minutes, or until soft, before blending.

Per Serving: Calories: 747; Saturated Fat: 7g; Total Fat: 43g; Protein: 19g; Total Carbs: 92g; Fiber: 23g; Sodium: 441mg

TURMERIC

Turmeric dates back almost 4,000 years in India. Both Ayurvedic and traditional Chinese medicine consider turmeric to be a digestive aid that can help reduce gas and bloating, and stimulate bile production in the liver, which helps the body break down fats efficiently. Because turmeric improves liver function, it is also a treatment for jaundice in both these healing traditions. Interestingly, the therapeutic actions of turmeric were not studied extensively by modern medicine until about 1970. Today, research has confirmed that turmeric is a healing remedy for various inflammatory diseases.

AT A GLANCE: curcumin, turmerone

HEALING POWER: The anti-inflammatory and antioxidant powers of turmeric can be attributed to curcumin, the ingredient that also gives the spice its notable color. Curcumin blocks several inflammatory pathways, reducing overall inflammation in the body. As an antioxidant, turmeric fights oxidative damage by neutralizing free radicals. It also enhances the activity of other antioxidants in the body, such as glutathione, and inhibits activation of certain inflammatory chemicals. Curcumin functions as a digestive aid, stimulating and enhancing the action of digestive enzymes. It also helps lower cholesterol and thin the blood. Turmerone, a component of turmeric's volatile oil, helps fight cancer by inhibiting cell proliferation. Note that the healing power of turmeric is enhanced when combined with black pepper.

HEALTH BENEFITS/MEDICAL CONDITIONS: Turmeric can help reduce swelling and may benefit those with rheumatoid arthritis or anyone with joint swelling. Topically, turmeric can be used for athlete's foot and psoriasis. It may also help with asthma and eczema. As a result of its cholesterol-lowering and blood-thinning effects, turmeric may reduce the risk of heart attack, stroke, and heart disease. The digestive powers of turmeric may help alleviate stomachache, gas, and bloating, which may benefit people with irritable bowel syndrome or other inflammatory bowel diseases. Turmeric may help prevent and fight cancer.

CONSUMPTION: ½ to 1 teaspoon, ground

TURMERIC GINGER TONIC

Serves 1

Prep time: 10 minutes

Reap the benefits of turmeric and ginger with this creamy, warm drink. These ingredients are two of the most widely studied ingredients in herbal medicine. They're used independently, and together, to fight a wide variety of issues. This tonic may help those with nausea, inflammation, and reduced immune function.

INGREDIENTS

1 cup unsweetened vanilla almond milk

1 teaspoon ground turmeric

1 teaspoon ground ginger

In a small saucepan over medium heat, whisk the almond milk, turmeric, and ginger to blend. Heat, stirring frequently, until warm.

INGREDIENT TIP

Turmeric stains very easily, so be careful with spills. If swapping ground turmeric for fresh turmeric root, add 1 tablespoon sliced fresh turmeric to the saucepan, bring the liquid to a boil. Let simmer for about 10 minutes, then strain out the turmeric pieces before drinking.

Per Serving: Calories: 54; Saturated Fat: 0g; Total Fat: 3g; Protein: 1g; Total Carbs: 5g; Fiber: 2g; Sodium: 181mg

BROCCOLI, GINGER, AND TURMERIC SOUP

Serves 4

Prep time: 15 minutes

Cook time: 30 minutes

This soup has *super* immunity-boosting powers (pun intended). Research shows that black pepper makes the compounds in turmeric about 2,000 percent more bioavailable, so you will get all the antioxidant effects from the spices and veggies! Enjoy this soup on its own, with 1 cup of whole grains, or serve it with a piece of warm sourdough bread.

INGREDIENTS

2 tablespoons extra-virgin olive oil

2 tablespoons roughly chopped peeled fresh ginger

2 leeks, cleaned well and finely chopped

2 broccoli heads, cut into florets

4 cups low-sodium vegetable stock

1 teaspoon ground turmeric

1 teaspoon salt

1 teaspoon freshly ground black pepper

1. In a large saucepan over medium heat, heat the olive oil. Add the ginger and cook for about 1 minute until fragrant.

2. Add the leeks and sauté for 3 minutes until lightly browned and softened.

3. Add the broccoli and sauté for 2 minutes until bright green.

4. Add the vegetable stock, turmeric, salt, and pepper. Bring the mixture to a simmer. Partially cover the pan and cook for 20 minutes, or until the broccoli is soft and fully cooked. Remove from the heat and let cool slightly.

5. Working in batches, transfer the soup to a blender or food processor and blend the soup until smooth. Return the blended soup to the pot and serve warm.

SUBSTITUTION TIP

You can substitute frozen leeks and broccoli for fresh, just increase the sauté time by 2 to 3 minutes for each ingredient to ensure they are fully cooked.

Per Serving: Calories: 174; Saturated Fat: 1g; Total Fat: 8g; Protein: 7g; Total Carbs: 23g; Fiber: 7g; Sodium: 671mg

GINGER

Ginger has been cultivated in India and China for thousands of years, where it is widely used for its curative properties, specifically for nausea. In Ayurvedic tradition, ginger is used to promote digestion, respiration, and relieve joint pain. The Greeks and Romans used the spice as a digestive aid. When the plant traveled to Europe, Queen Elizabeth I had gingerbread men cooked for her guests!

AT A GLANCE: gingerol, shogaol

HEALING POWER: Gingerol, the main active compound in ginger, helps quell nausea, as well as indigestion. Gingerol is also a powerful anti-inflammatory that reduces swelling and can improve joint pain and stiffness. The pungent herb provides a warming sensation, which can ease breathing and improve cold and cough symptoms. Gingerol, and another powerful constituent of the root, shogaol, have antioxidant effects that may help protect against cancer and fight free radicals in the body. Ginger has cardioprotective elements that help lower lipids, stimulate circulation, and prevent blood clots.

HEALTH BENEFITS/MEDICAL CONDITIONS: Thanks to gingerol's powerful antinausea effects, ginger is a good antidote for nausea, vomiting, and indigestion. Ginger may be helpful for pregnant women who struggle with nausea and vomiting, and for anyone who suffers from motion sickness or upset stomach. It can also be used to promote digestion, which may help relieve heartburn. Ginger provides antioxidants that can help protect against cancer. The anti-inflammatory powers of ginger are helpful for those with rheumatoid arthritis, osteoarthritis, and joint pain. Ginger may provide effective nausea and pain relief for those with migraines and headaches. The warming action of ginger in the body, as well as its antiviral effects, may help fight off cold and flu.

CONSUMPTION: 1 teaspoon dried or 2 teaspoons fresh

KALE GINGER SMOOTHIE

Serves 1

Prep time: 5 minutes

Detox is the name of the game with this green smoothie. Ginger and kale combine to create a delicious and nutritious elixir. The chia seeds and flaxseed can help combat constipation by moving things along. I recommend blending this smoothie to reset digestion after an indulgent time like the holidays.

INGREDIENTS

2 cups stemmed kale leaf pieces

1 cup unsweetened vanilla almond milk

½ banana, peeled and frozen

½ cup frozen blueberries

1 tablespoon chia seeds

1 tablespoon ground flaxseed

2 teaspoons grated peeled fresh ginger

¼ teaspoon ground cinnamon

3 or 4 ice cubes (optional)

In a high-speed blender, combine the kale, almond milk, banana, blueberries, chia seeds, flaxseed, ginger, cinnamon, and ice (if using). Blend on high speed until smooth.

STORAGE TIP

Make blending smoothies easier with pre-mixed single-serve bags. Combine all of the ingredients (except the almond milk) in single serving bags or plastic containers and store them in the freezer. When you want to enjoy a smoothie, blend the contents of 1 bag with 1 cup of almond milk.

Per Serving: Calories: 330; Saturated Fat: 1g; Total Fat: 12g; Protein: 11g; Total Carbs: 49g; Fiber: 15g; Sodium: 241mg

APPLE CINNAMON GINGER OATS

Serves 1

Prep time: 10 minutes

Cook time: 35 minutes

Elevate your ordinary bowl of oats with some spice! Fresh ginger complements the cinnamon and nutmeg here and blends nicely with the creamy oats. This recipe is incredibly grounding and is great for breakfast or whenever you feel under the weather.

INGREDIENTS

1 cup unsweetened plain almond milk

¼ cup steel cut oats

1 apple, chopped

1 tablespoon finely grated peeled fresh ginger

1 teaspoon ground cinnamon

½ teaspoon ground nutmeg

¼ cup chopped walnuts

1. In a saucepan over medium heat, bring the almond milk to a boil, then stir in the oats.

2. Reduce the heat to low and cook for 25 to 30 minutes, stirring occasionally, until the oats are your desired texture.

3. Stir in the apple, ginger, cinnamon, and nutmeg. To serve, top with the walnuts.

SUBSTITUTION TIP

If you don't have fresh ginger, substitute ¼ teaspoon ground ginger. You can use quick-cooking oats, if you prefer. Nutritionally, quick cook oats and steel cut oats are similar, but the quick-cooking are technically more processed. The quick-cooking oats are steamed, rolled (made into old-fashioned oats), and then cut into smaller pieces for faster cooking.

Per Serving: Calories: 577; Saturated Fat: 3g; Total Fat: 30g; Protein: 13g; Total Carbs: 66g; Fiber: 16g; Sodium: 365mg

CUMIN

Native to Egypt, cumin seeds were used widely as a medicinal herb in ancient Egypt to treat coughs, rotten teeth, and stomachaches. In Indian culture, cumin is used as a remedy for everything from insomnia to fevers and scorpion stings. The spicy, earthy taste of cumin is distinct, and provides various healing benefits as well as a depth of flavor for dishes such as chili and curry.

AT A GLANCE: cuminaldehyde, fiber, iron

HEALING POWER: Cumin seeds are a great source of dietary fiber and iron. Cumin also has antioxidant, anti-inflammatory, antimicrobial, and antidiabetic effects in the body. Cumin is a digestive aid that stimulates pancreatic enzymes, helping promote optimal digestion of foods and assimilation of nutrients. The main constituent in cumin, cuminaldehyde, helps fight disease through its antimicrobial power and may help improve blood sugar control.

HEALTH BENEFITS/MEDICAL CONDITIONS: Cumin is a great source of iron, which can be helpful for iron deficiency and anemia. Cumin promotes optimal digestion and may be helpful for those with irritable bowel syndrome. Cumin may help promote blood sugar control, which benefits people with diabetes. Cumin can ease the effects of diabetes in other ways as well. It has been shown to help reduce the amount of advanced glycation end products (AGEs) in the bloodstream, which can cause damage to the kidneys, eyes, and blood vessels. Cumin also has anti-inflammatory effects, which may protect against cancer and reduce overall inflammation levels in the body.

CONSUMPTION: 1 to 2 teaspoons

THREE-BEAN SLOW COOKER CHILI

Serves 8

Prep time: 20 minutes

Cook time: 4 hours

There's nothing like a warm bowl of chili on a cold winter day. This simple, slow cooker soup has all the benefits of complex carbohydrate–rich beans and antioxidant-filled spices, without the typical high fat and sodium content of chili. Making soup at home allows you to control what goes into it, especially salt. Using flavorful alternatives, such as onion, garlic, and spices, is a simple way to season soup with extra healing benefits!

INGREDIENTS

2 (15-ounce) cans kidney beans, drained and rinsed

1 (15-ounce) can black beans, drained and rinsed

1 (15-ounce) can pinto beans, drained and rinsed

1 (15-ounce) can diced tomatoes

2½ cups low-sodium vegetable stock

1 green bell pepper, chopped

1 white onion, chopped

2 garlic cloves, finely minced

1 teaspoon ground cumin

1 teaspoon cayenne pepper

1. In a 5-quart slow cooker, combine the kidney beans, black beans, pinto beans, tomatoes and their juices, vegetable stock, green bell pepper, onion, garlic, cumin, and cayenne. Stir to combine.

2. Cover the cooker and cook on high heat for 4 hours.

VARIATION TIP

Serve with chopped scallion. To make the chili spicier, stir in 1 chopped chile pepper of choice, such as a jalapeño.

Per Serving: Calories: 269; Saturated Fat: 0g; Total Fat: 1g; Protein: 17g; Total Carbs: 50g; Fiber: 16g; Sodium: 67mg

CREAMY LIME DRESSING

Serves 6

Prep time: 5 minutes

This tangy dressing is great for salads and grain bowls. The cumin adds flavor dimension to this nutrient-packed green blend. Drizzle the dressing on a crunchy romaine lettuce salad or try it on the Brown Rice Bowl (page 104)!

INGREDIENTS

1 bunch fresh cilantro, roughly chopped

½ cup extra-virgin olive oil

½ avocado, peeled and pitted

Juice of 1 lime

1 garlic clove, peeled

¼ teaspoon ground cumin

Salt

Freshly ground black pepper

In a high-speed blender, combine the cilantro, olive oil, avocado, lime juice, garlic, and cumin. Blend until smooth, adding water, 1 tablespoon at a time, to achieve your desired consistency. Taste and season with salt and pepper.

STORAGE TIP

Embrace sustainability! Recycle your used glass containers (mustard jars, nut butter containers, etc.) and use them to store salad dressings. You can also buy spices loose, in bulk, and store them in glass jars at home.

Per Serving: Calories: 174; Saturated Fat: 3g; Total Fat: 19g; Protein: 1g; Total Carbs: 3g; Fiber: 2g; Sodium: 32mg

CAYENNE

Cayenne pepper is a type of chile pepper known for its very hot taste. The peppers are dried and ground to make a powerful spice that has been used medicinally in Chinese and Ayurvedic traditions as a warming circulatory stimulant. Capsaicin, an active component of chile peppers, is widely celebrated as a metabolism booster, but note that research shows the effect is small and if you consume cayenne regularly, the body can build up a tolerance. Don't worry, spice lovers! There are many healing properties of cayenne.

AT A GLANCE: capsaicin, carotenoids

HEALING POWER: The active ingredient in cayenne, capsaicin, is known to have analgesic powers that can provide pain relief and boost metabolism. When used externally, cayenne can desensitize nerves that cause pain. Internally, cayenne can stimulate the secretion of digestive enzymes that improve digestion. Cayenne may increase circulation, which causes the body to burn more calories, and may promote weight loss. Cayenne peppers also contain carotenoids that work as antioxidants in the body, protecting cells and tissues from oxidative damage.

HEALTH BENEFITS/MEDICAL CONDITIONS: The antioxidant and capsaicin content in cayenne peppers may protect against and prevent cancer. Capsaicin has potent pain-relieving properties and may help people with muscle spasms or joint pain. It may also be helpful for those with arthritis or sports-related injuries, as it may increase circulation. Capsaicin may boost metabolism and decrease appetite, which is beneficial for weight loss. Cayenne can be used as a digestive aid and may ease digestive woes, such as gas. Cayenne can be used to ease sore throats and provide relief from congestion, coughs, and cold.

CONSUMPTION: 1 teaspoon

FIERY HUMMUS

Serves 6

Prep time: 15 minutes

Cayenne certainly kicks this hummus up a notch! The antioxidant-rich spice adds a fiery flare to the garlicky dip. You can control how much—or how little—spice you want by starting with ¼ teaspoon of cayenne and taste-testing before adding more. Serve the hummus with carrots and celery, or for even more spice, sliced peppers!

INGREDIENTS

1 (15-ounce) can no-salt-added chickpeas, drained and rinsed

3 tablespoons extra-virgin olive oil

2 tablespoons tahini

Juice of ½ lemon

1 garlic clove, crushed

1 teaspoon ground cumin

1 teaspoon ground coriander

¼ teaspoon ground cayenne pepper

Salt

Freshly ground black pepper

In a food processor or blender, combine the chickpeas, olive oil, tahini, lemon juice, garlic, cumin, coriander, and cayenne. Process until smooth. Taste and season with salt and black pepper.

VARIATION TIP

You can leave out the cumin and coriander if you prefer a simple lemon-based hummus.

Per Serving: Calories: 123; Saturated Fat: 1g; Total Fat: 10g; Protein: 3g; Total Carbs: 7g; Fiber: 1g; Sodium: 89mg

SPICY POTATO WEDGES

Serves 3

Prep time: 15 minutes

Cook time: 25 minutes

This easy, spicy alternative to French fries will boost your metabolism and help promote digestion. You can use any variety of sweet potato or white potato, but russet potatoes tend to produce the best consistency. Be sure to buy organic potatoes and scrub the skins well. Potato skin has a ton of fiber and vitamins, so be sure to eat the skin, too.

INGREDIENTS

3 large potatoes, cut into wedges

¼ cup extra-virgin olive oil

2 garlic cloves, finely minced

½ teaspoon paprika

¼ teaspoon sea salt

⅛ teaspoon ground cayenne pepper

1. Preheat the oven to 450°F. Line a baking sheet with parchment paper and set aside.

2. In a large bowl, toss together the potatoes, olive oil, garlic, paprika, salt, and cayenne until well coated. Transfer the potatoes to the prepared baking sheet, spreading them into an even layer.

3. Roast for 25 minutes, turning every 10 minutes, until nicely browned.

VARIATION TIP

Make the potato wedges sweet (but still spicy)! Swap the olive oil for coconut oil and skip the garlic and paprika. Add 1 teaspoon ground cinnamon.

Per Serving: Calories: 403; Saturated Fat: 3g; Total Fat: 17g; Protein: 6g; Total Carbs: 59g; Fiber: 9g; Sodium: 179mg

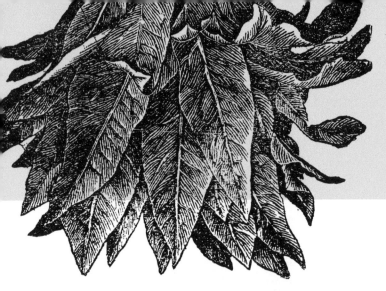

TIPS AND TRICKS TO SKIP THE GARLIC SMELL

Love cooking with garlic, but hate the garlic smell? Here are some tips on how to remove the garlic cloves from their papery skins efficiently without stinking for days after (although garlic can be used as an effective bug spray)! Break the head into cloves and place the cloves in a glass jar. Shake the glass jar vigorously for 15 to 30 seconds, then pull out the cloves. The papery skins should come off easily—and voilà, you have peeled garlic. To get the garlic smell off your hands, rinse your hands under cold water while rubbing your fingers over something made of stainless steel, like a spoon or bowl. If you don't have dry skin or any cuts on your hands, you can also use lemon juice, toothpaste, or mouthwash as a hand wash in place of the stainless steel.

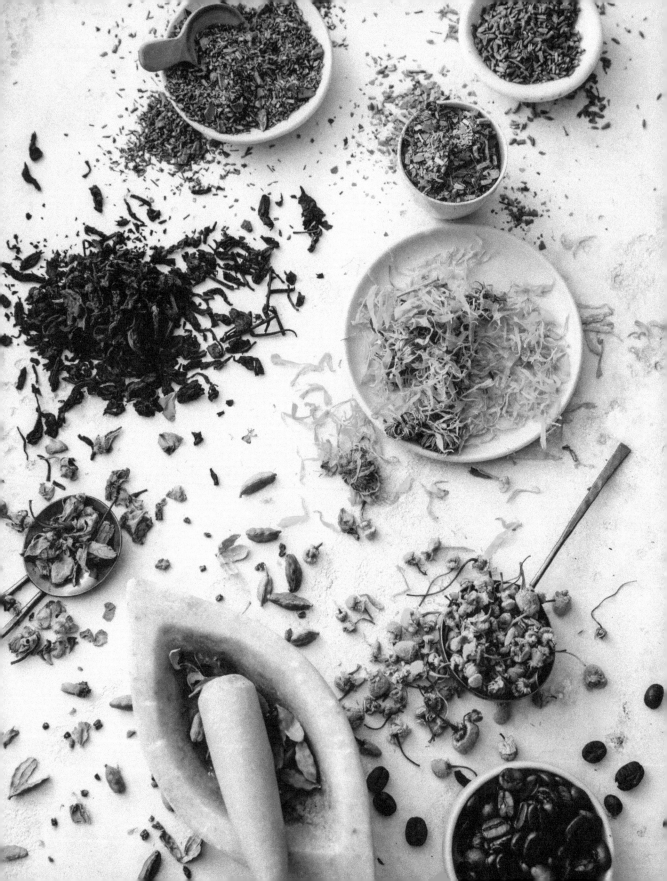

7

Coffee and Tea

Coffee and tea are among the most widely consumed beverages worldwide. Whether you're looking for a caffeine boost in the morning or a soothing warm beverage before bed, coffee and tea can provide various options, all with lots of nutritional and healing benefits. This chapter explores coffee, then jumps into traditional and herbal tisanes, or infusions. Finally, you'll read about traditional teas, including green tea and oolong varieties from the *Camellia sinensis* plant, as well as herbal yerba mate and rooibos. Bottoms up!

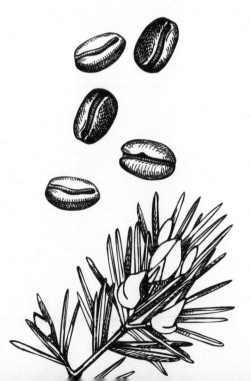

COFFEE

If you're like many people, you start your day with a delicious (and caffeinating) cup of coffee. According to the National Coffee Association, 63 percent of American adults drink coffee daily. Coffee has been used medicinally as a stimulant and energy booster in various cultures, helping people feel less tired and improve their mood and their physical performance. Caffeine, the stimulant in coffee, is considered the most popular drug in the world!

AT A GLANCE: B vitamins, caffeine, chlorogenic acids

HEALING POWER: The caffeine in coffee is an incredible central nervous system stimulant. It can promote alertness and improve mood. Coffee is a diuretic that increases gastric motility (contractions of the smooth muscle in the gastrointestinal tract) and intestinal peristalsis (wavelike movement of intestinal muscle). Coffee is a good source of various energy-promoting B vitamins such as riboflavin, pantothenic acid, and niacin. The chlorogenic acid in coffee is a key antioxidant that helps fight damage from free radicals. Coffee is also used topically in skin products to reduce inflammation and promote blood flow to the area, especially with cellulite or under-eye bags.

HEALTH BENEFITS/MEDICAL CONDITIONS: The caffeine in coffee can improve energy levels, fight fatigue, and improve mood. Athletes may see improved performance with caffeine. The diuretic- and digestion-promoting qualities of coffee may be helpful for those with constipation. Caffeine may boost a person's metabolic rate and result in weight loss. Caffeine is a bronchodilator that helps open the airways in the lungs and may be beneficial for those with asthma. Coffee is the largest source of antioxidants in the Western diet and may help protect against cancer. Coffee may reduce the risk of neurodegenerative diseases, such as Alzheimer's and Parkinson's diseases.

CONSUMPTION: 8 to 16 ounces

COFFEE OAT SMOOTHIE

Serves 1

Prep time: 5 minutes

This creamy, sweet blend combines two of my favorite morning ingredients: coffee and oats. I like to think of it as morning in a cup: It has my coffee, banana, oats, and almond butter all blended into one delicious drink. Though it can be a caffeine and complex carbohydrate–rich boost first thing in the morning, this smoothie is a great pick-me-up any time of day!

INGREDIENTS

½ cup brewed coffee, cooled

½ cup unsweetened plain almond milk

½ banana, peeled and frozen

¼ cup old-fashioned rolled oats

1 tablespoon almond butter

3 or 4 ice cubes

In a high-speed blender, combine the coffee, almond milk, banana, oats, almond butter, and ice. Blend on high speed until smooth.

VARIATION TIP

Looking to improve digestion? Swap the almond butter for 1 tablespoon each of flaxseed and chia seeds.

Per Serving: Calories: 269; Saturated Fat: 1g; Total Fat: 14g; Protein: 8g; Total Carbs: 31g; Fiber: 6g; Sodium: 185mg

GREEN TEA

Green tea, like black and oolong teas, comes from the *Camellia sinensis* plant. The variations among types of teas are due to their preparation. Black tea is fully fermented and oxidized, whereas oolong is only fermented and partially oxidized. In general, green tea is not fermented, or is only allowed to ferment for a short time. This minimal processing means green tea contains the most polyphenols of all varieties. This antioxidant-filled beverage has been used as an anti-inflammatory and stimulating medicinal tonic for centuries in traditional Chinese medicine. Matcha is a type of green tea celebrated for its amplified antioxidants and caffeine.

AT A GLANCE: caffeine, epigallocatechin gallate (EGCG), L-theanine

HEALING POWER: EGCG is one of the most studied and powerful compounds in green tea. EGCG is an antioxidant that prevents cell damage by fending off harmful free radicals. Green tea contains caffeine, which acts as a stimulant in the body. With less caffeine than coffee, tea boosts the mood without extra jitters. In green tea, EGCG and caffeine combine to increase fat oxidation (fat burning) and boost metabolic rate. EGCG also works to effectively lower cholesterol in the body. L-theanine, a relaxation-inducing amino acid in green tea, is responsible for the tea's specific taste and helps increase brain function. L-theanine may increase serotonin, dopamine, and GABA levels, improving mood and cognitive function.

HEALTH BENEFITS/MEDICAL CONDITIONS: The antioxidant effects of EGCG may reduce the risk of cancer and decrease overall inflammation in the body. Green tea may boost metabolism and increase the rate of fat burning, which can promote weight loss and prevent obesity. The caffeine in green tea may boost mood, athletic performance, and increase alertness. Green tea may improve cognitive function and memory. EGCG in green tea may lower cholesterol, which leads to improved heart health and reduces the risk of stroke. Although it contains caffeine (a natural diuretic), green tea is a hydrating beverage that can improve overall bodily function and fluid status.

CONSUMPTION: 8 to 16 ounces, brewed

MATCHA SMOOTHIE

Serves 1

Prep time: 5 minutes

I'm not a huge fan of traditional hot matcha, but I absolutely love a matcha smoothie. Matcha boosts the antioxidant healing power of a simple green smoothie with its high EGCG content and lends a delicious, crisp taste. Green tea is typically fairly astringent and aromatic, but the banana and unsweetened vanilla almond milk help mellow the flavor (and slightly sweeten it) so you can sip happily.

INGREDIENTS

1 cup fresh spinach

¾ cup unsweetened vanilla almond milk

1 banana, peeled and frozen

1 tablespoon chia seeds

1 tablespoon ground flaxseed

1 teaspoon matcha powder

3 or 4 ice cubes (optional)

In a high-speed blender, combine the spinach, almond milk, banana, chia seeds, flaxseed, matcha powder, and ice (if using). Blend on high speed until smooth.

INGREDIENT TIP

Do your research and find a high-quality source of matcha. Bitter-tasting matcha may mean it's a lower quality product. You want the matcha you purchase to be from Japan, with a vibrant, bright green color.

Per Serving: Calories: 274; Saturated Fat: 1g; Total Fat: 12g; Protein: 8g; Total Carbs: 39g; Fiber: 13g; Sodium: 162mg

OOLONG

Made from the *Camellia sinensis* plant, oolong is a fruity tea at the midpoint between traditional black and green teas in taste, color, and oxidation. Native to the Wuyi Mountain region of China, oolong has been used for centuries to regulate body temperature, promote digestion, and prevent tooth decay and skin irritations. Note that tea, in general, including oolong and green varietals, may reduce absorption of iron from plant foods. Adding lemon, a source of vitamin C, to your tea can help mitigate this minor effect and increase iron absorption.

AT A GLANCE: caffeine, epigallocatechin gallate (EGCG), theaflavins

HEALING POWER: Oolong contains the powerful polyphenol, EGCG, which has many functions in the body. The primary function of EGCG is as an antioxidant, fighting free radical damage in the body and preventing oxidative stress. Oolong's active ingredients reduce inflammation in the body, help reduce blood sugar levels, and improve insulin sensitivity. The antioxidants may also improve heart health, as tea consumption has been shown to reduce the risk of hypertension. Oolong contains theaflavins and theanine, which may help reduce oxidative stress, promote feelings of relaxation, and provide neuroprotective effects. Oolong was historically used to prevent tooth decay, and it has been shown to reduce dental plaque.

HEALTH BENEFITS/MEDICAL CONDITIONS: Oolong also has active ingredients, including antioxidants, that fight obesity, diabetes, atherosclerosis, heart disease, and hypertension. The caffeine and theaflavins in oolong may boost mood, increase alertness, improve overall brain function, and prevent cognitive diseases, such as Alzheimer's and Parkinson's diseases. Oolong may promote optimal dental health.

CONSUMPTION: 8 to 16 ounces, brewed

ICED RASPBERRY OOLONG TEA

Serves 2

Prep time: 10 minutes, plus cooling time

Oolong tea is sometimes described as the middle of the road between black and green tea. It's not as rich as black tea, but more processed than green tea. Raspberries complement the oolong taste and provide a bit of tang and sweetness in this refreshing drink.

INGREDIENTS

2 cups water

1 cup frozen raspberries

2 oolong tea bags

2 lemon wedges (optional)

Honey (optional)

Ice

1. In a small saucepan over high heat, bring the water to a boil. Add the raspberries and tea bags. Remove from the heat, cover the pan, and steep for 3 to 5 minutes.

2. Remove the tea bags and strain the raspberries from the tea using a fine-mesh sieve set over a bowl or pitcher.

3. Stir in the lemon juice (if using) and honey (if using), then let cool. Serve over ice.

INGREDIENT TIP

Reserve the oolong-infused raspberries and make oolong raspberry chia jam. Mix the strained raspberries with 2 tablespoons chia seeds, 1 tablespoon freshly squeezed lemon juice, and 1 tablespoon maple syrup. Transfer to a glass jar and refrigerate for at least 2 hours before using.

Per Serving: Calories: 7; Saturated Fat: 0g; Total Fat: 0g; Protein: 0g; Total Carbs: 2g; Fiber: 0g; Sodium: 0mg

YERBA MATE

Made from an infusion of the leaves of the *Ilex paraguariensis* tree, yerba mate is a traditional beverage of the Guaraní people of South America. This caffeinating beverage plays a social role in South American culture, where people are thought to drink more than 1 liter of yerba mate per day. The tea is traditionally consumed as part of daily custom and for an energy boost, rather than for its medicinal qualities, but it is an antioxidant powerhouse with many health-promoting properties.

AT A GLANCE: caffeine, chlorogenic acid, saponins

HEALING POWER: Yerba mate contains less caffeine than coffee but more than black tea. It isn't acidic like coffee, so it may be a good alternative for those with acid reflux. The caffeine in yerba mate can boost energy levels and improve focus. Yerba mate contains various polyphenols, including chlorogenic acid, which provide powerful antioxidant protection. The distinct flavor of mate can be attributed to saponins, which are known for their anti-inflammatory and cholesterol-lowering effects. The tea may reduce appetite and boost metabolism, leading to weight loss. Yerba mate can help improve insulin signaling and promote normal blood sugar levels (as long as you're not adding a ton of sugar to the drink)!

HEALTH BENEFITS/MEDICAL CONDITIONS: The caffeine in yerba mate may promote brain function, improve mental alertness, and boost energy. The caffeine may also improve physical performance in athletes. The metabolism-boosting effects of caffeine and filling fluid content of yerba mate may promote weight loss. The antimicrobial effects of yerba mate may boost the immune system and prevent infection. Yerba mate contains large amounts of antioxidants, such as chlorogenic acid, which may protect against cancer. The saponins in yerba mate may help lower cholesterol levels, promoting optimal heart health.

CONSUMPTION: 8 to 16 ounces, brewed

YERBA MATE COCONUT LATTE

Serves 1

Prep time: 10 minutes

Deliciously warm and indulgent, this yerba mate coconut latte will keep you pleasantly caffeinated without the jitters from coffee. Coconut milk is high in medium-chain triglycerides, which may promote weight loss when used in small quantities (given that it is high in calories). Its creamy, nutty taste complements the chocolate-like flavor of the yerba mate.

INGREDIENTS

1 cup water

2 tablespoons full-fat coconut milk

½ teaspoon ground cinnamon

⅛ teaspoon vanilla extract

1 yerba mate tea bag

In a small saucepan over high heat, combine the water, coconut milk, cinnamon, and vanilla. Bring to a boil. Remove from the heat, add the tea bag, and steep for 3 to 5 minutes. Remove and discard the tea bag and serve warm.

SUBSTITUTION TIP

The full-fat coconut milk adds an indulgent creaminess, but you can swap the coconut milk for unsweetened plain almond milk, or any other nut-based milk, if desired.

Per Serving: Calories: 62; Saturated Fat: 6g; Total Fat: 6g; Protein: 1g; Total Carbs: 2g; Fiber: 1g; Sodium: 4mg

ROOIBOS

Rooibos, a part of the *Aspalathus linearis* plant native to South Africa, is a caffeine-free herbal tea. However, it's not technically a tea, but rather an herbal tisane made by using the plant's leaves to create an infusion. Rooibos has been used in South African culture for many years to soothe colicky babies, promote relaxation, and ease stomach cramps. Today, rooibos is widely consumed as a caffeine-free alternative to black and green teas.

AT A GLANCE: aspalalinin, aspalathin, nothofagin

HEALING POWER: Rooibos contains potent antioxidants, aspalathin and aspalalinin, that help fight free radicals in the body. It also contains the antioxidant nothofagin, which has been shown to inhibit inflammation caused by high blood sugar. The greatest healing power of rooibos comes from these antioxidants, which promote general health and reduce the risk of chronic diseases. Consuming rooibos has been shown to decrease cholesterol and triglyceride levels, reducing the risk of cardiovascular disease. Rooibos is a caffeine-free tea, meaning it will not act as a stimulant in the body, and can help promote relaxation.

HEALTH BENEFITS/MEDICAL CONDITIONS: Rooibos is a good option for people who are looking to avoid or limit caffeine, including those who suffer from insomnia or heart problems, or who are pregnant. The antioxidant power of aspalathin in rooibos may protect against cancer and cardiovascular disease. Rooibos may promote heart health through the reduction of cholesterol and triglycerides. The antioxidant activity of aspalathin and nothofagin in rooibos may reduce inflammation and prevent complications from diabetes.

CONSUMPTION: 8 to 16 ounces, brewed

HOT ROOIBOS APPLE CIDER

Serves 2

Prep time: 15 minutes

Sip yourself to sleep with this deliciously warm rooibos cider. This sweet, seasonal blend is a great after-dinner treat with some sweetness and a bit of spice. The combination of rooibos and the warm cider is incredibly satisfying and a great immune system booster.

INGREDIENTS

1 cup water

1 cup apple juice or apple cider (no sugar added, organic)

2 tablespoons freshly squeezed lemon juice

¼ teaspoon ground cinnamon

⅛ teaspoon ground ginger

2 rooibos tea bags

In a small saucepan over medium heat, combine the water, apple juice, lemon juice, cinnamon, and ginger. Bring to a simmer, then remove from the heat and add the tea bags. Steep for 10 minutes. Remove and discard the tea bags and serve warm.

INGREDIENT TIP

I don't generally recommend purchasing bottled juice but, once in a while, an organic, unsweetened juice is a delicious treat.
Look for a juice with the fewest ingredients (ideally only the fruit, like apples) and no added sugars.

Per Serving: Calories: 61; Saturated Fat: 0g; Total Fat: 0g; Protein: 0g; Total Carbs: 15g; Fiber: 1g; Sodium: 8mg

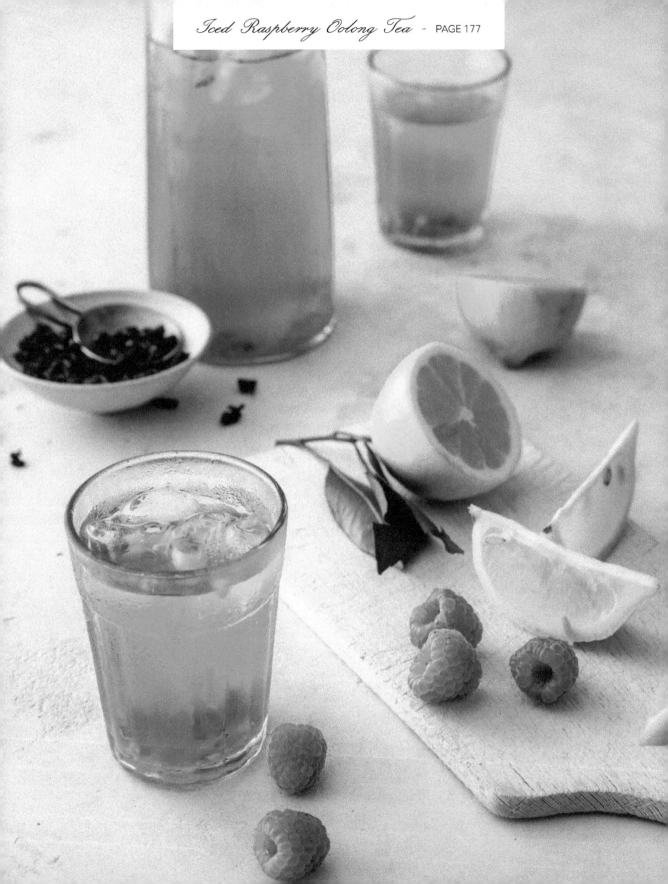

Iced Raspberry Oolong Tea - PAGE 177

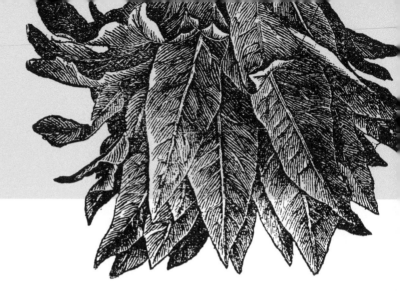

THE TRUTH ABOUT DECAF

Decaf drinkers beware! Decaffein-ated coffee or tea doesn't actually contain zero caffeine. According to the Mayo Clinic, one 8-ounce cup of decaf coffee or tea contains 2 to 5 milligrams of caffeine. Although this amount is much less than the caffeine-filled regular versions, it isn't completely devoid of the stimulant. Plus, actual caffeine content depends on the processing method and quality of the bean. Decaffeinated coffee is generally made using a solvent to extract or dissolve the caffeine. This process used to be of concern, as the chemical solvent used was benzene, a carcinogenic ingredient. Though the process is much safer now, there are still chemicals involved. If you choose decaf, try to go organic, as coffee beans tend to be a large source of mold. You may be better off choosing a naturally caffeine-free herbal tea!

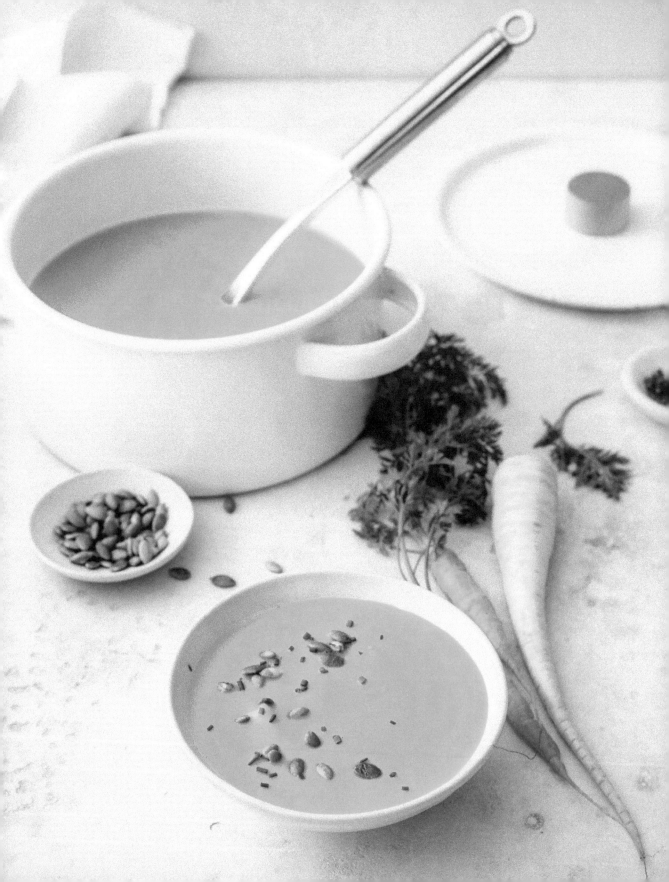

RESOURCES

WEBSITES AND APPS

Center for Science in the Public Interest

The Center for Science in the Public Interest (CSPI) provides great resources for independent science-backed advice, especially with regard to food dyes, sweeteners, and other food additives. CSPI has a great ranking of food additives and a glossary of the chemicals used to flavor and preserve food. https://cspinet.org/

Environmental Working Group's Shopper's Guide to Pesticides in Produce: Dirty Dozen™ and Clean Fifteen™ Lists

The Environmental Working Group has created lists to guide you in purchasing produce grown with the fewest pesticides possible. If you are unable to purchase everything organic, use these lists to prioritize which organic produce to buy. Avoid the Dirty Dozen fruits and vegetables or buy them only as organic, and purchase the Clean Fifteen as conventionally grown. www.ewg.org/foodnews/

Environmental Working Group's Healthy Living App

The Environmental Working Group's Healthy Living app is a great supermarket tool to help you select the healthiest products, cosmetics, and sunscreen. This app allows you to scan a barcode or browse through lists of products and it will alert you to any ingredient, nutrition, or processing concerns, and provide recommendations for alternatives.

Harvest App

Use the Harvest App to see what produce is in season in your area. The app will give you tips on how to select and store each item. The app also provides guidance on pesticide levels of certain fruits and vegetables, giving them a green, yellow, or red rating to help guide your choices.

BOOKS

Hari, Vani. *The Food Babe Way: Break Free from the Hidden Toxins in Your Food and Lose Weight, Look Years Younger, and Get Healthy in Just 21 Days!*
Vani Hari provides ample insight into what is really in your food, especially regarding toxins. She provides helpful guidance on how to decipher and decode ingredient labels, sheds light on the food industry, and speaks more in depth about GMOs.

Lipman, Frank. *How to Be Well: The 6 Keys to a Happy Life*
Dr. Frank Lipman is a physician who is knowledgeable in both Eastern and Western approaches to medicine. His book is a treasure trove of healthy living tips, offering a wide range of highly informative tidbits on how to live a healthy lifestyle.

Ottolenghi, Yotam. *Ottolenghi Simple: A Cookbook*
If you're looking for a delicious way to cook vegetables, *Ottolenghi Simple* is an amazing resource. This cookbook offers 130 flavor-packed recipes that can be made in 30 minutes or less, with 10 or fewer ingredients, and everything is centered on fresh produce.

Pitchford, Paul. *Healing with Whole Foods: Asian Traditions and Modern Nutrition.*
Paul Pitchford's book, *Healing with Whole Foods* is the bible for mixing modern and ancient traditions concerning lifestyle and nutrition. This book is a great resource for learning more about traditional Chinese medicine and the ways you can incorporate the practices into your daily life.

Yeager, Selene, and the Editors of *Prevention. The Doctors Book of Food Remedies: The Latest Findings on the Power of Food to Treat and Prevent Health Problems—From Aging and Diabetes to Ulcers and Yeast Infections*
This book is a great resource for those looking for additional research-backed information about food remedies. The book provides profiles based on specific foods and health concerns, as well as helpful tips from doctors.

REFERENCES

AANMC. "Kale 101: The Naturopathic Kitchen." Association of Accredited Naturopathic Colleges. Accessed October 7, 2019. https://tryl2012.blogspot.com/2019/01/kale-101-naturopathic-kitchen.html.

Adams, Ken, and Dan Drost. "Fennel in the Garden." Utah State University Cooperative Extension. March 2012. Accessed October 7, 2019. https://digitalcommons.usu.edu/cgi/viewcontent.cgi?referer=https://www.google.com/&httpsredir=1&article=1267&context=extension_curall.

Aghajanpour, Mohammad, Mohamad Reza Nazer, Zia Obeidavi, Mohsen Akbari, Parya Ezati, and Nasroallah Moradi Kor. "Functional Foods and Their Role in Cancer Prevention and Health Promotion: A Comprehensive Review." *American Journal of Cancer Research*. 7, no. 4 (2017): 740–769. www.ncbi.nlm.nih.gov/pmc/articles/PMC5411786/.

Ahmad, Zeeshan. "The Uses and Properties of Almond Oil." *Complementary Therapies in Clinical Practice* 16, no. 1 (2010): 10–12. https://doi.org/10.1016/j.ctcp.2009.06.015.

Akram, M., Ibrahim Shah, Khan Usmanghan, E. Mohiuddin, Abdul Sami, M. Asif, S. M. Ali Shah, et al. "*Zingiber officinale* Roscoe: A Medicinal Plant." *Pakistan Journal of Nutrition* 10, no. 4 (2011): 399–400. www.researchgate.net/profile/Muhammad_Akram60/publication/267378289_Zingiber_officinale_Roscoe_A_Medicinal_Plant/links/55e1217a08aecb1a7cc61a9a/Zingiber-officinale-Roscoe-A-Medicinal-Plant.pdf.

Auborn, Karen, Saijun Fan, Elliot Rosen, Leslie Goodwin, Alamelu Chandraskaren, David Williams, DaZhi Chen, et al. "Indole-3-Carbinol Is a Negative Regulator of Estrogen." *The Journal of Nutrition* 133, no. 7 (2003): 2470S–2475S. https://academic.oup.com/jn/article/133/7/2470S/4688465/.

Baranski, Marcin, Dominika Srednicka-Tober, Nikolaos Volakakis, et al. "Higher Antioxidant and Lower Cadmium Concentrations and Lower Incidence of Pesticide Residues in Organically Grown Crops: A Systematic Literature Review and Meta-Analyses." *British Journal of Nutrition* 112, no. 5 (2014): 794–811. doi:10.1017/S0007114514001366.

Bauman, Hannah, and Becky Nichols. "Food as Medicine: Watermelon (*Citrullus lanatus*, Cucurbitaceae)." American Botanical Council. Accessed October 8, 2019. http://cms .herbalgram.org/heg/volume12/07July/FaM_Watermelon.html?ts=1570583329 &signature=675a0ab8607e9551bc99b90735c51954.

Bauman, Hannah, and Taylor Moyer. "Food as Medicine: Avocado (*Persea americana*, Lauraceae)." American Botanical Council. June 2017. Accessed October 9, 2019. http://cms.herbalgram.org/heg/volume14/06June/FoodasMedicine_Avocado.html?ts =1570629264&signature=4edb29d2d8d913e6e6cff97fa4755485.

Bayan, Leyla, Peir Hossain Koulivand, and Ali Gorji. "Garlic: A Review of Potential Therapeutic Effects." *Avicenna Journal of Phytomedicine* 4, no. 1 (2014): 1–14. www.ncbi.nlm.nih .gov/pmc/articles/PMC4103721/.

Bhowmik, Debjit, K. P. Sampath Kumar, Shravan Paswan, and Shweta Srivastava. "Tomato–A Natural Medicine and Its Health Benefits." *Journal of Pharmacognosy and Phytochemistry* 1, no. 1 (2012): 24–28. www.researchgate.net/publication/285176270 _Tomato-A_Natural_Medicine_and_Its_Health_Benefits_INTRODUCTION_Tomatoes _are_a_member_of.

Biswas, Saibal K., Danny McClure, Luis A. Jimenez, Ian L. Megson, and Irfan Rahman. "Curcumin Induces Glutathione Biosynthesis and Inhibits NF-kB Activation and Interleukin-8 Release in Alveolar Epithelial Cells: Mechanism of Free Radical Scavenging Activity." *Antioxidant & Redox Signaling* 7, nos. 1–2 (2004). doi:10.1089/ars.2005.7.32.

Blondeau, Nicolas, Robert Lipsky, Miled Bourourou, Mark Duncan, Philip Gorelick, and Ann Marini. "Alpha-Linolenic Acid: An Omega-3 Fatty Acid with Neuroprotective Properties—Ready for Use in the Stroke Clinic?" *BioMed Research International* 2015. doi:10.1155/2015/519830.

Boyer, Jeanelle, and Rui Jai Lui. "Apple Phytochemicals and Their Health Benefits." *Nutrition Journal* 3, no. 5 (2004): 1–15. www.ncbi.nlm.nih.gov/pmc/articles/PMC442131 /pdf/1475-2891-3-5.pdf.

Camargo, Camila, Maria Christina C. Gomes-Marcondes, Nathalie Wutzki, and Hiroshi Aoyama. "Naringin Inhibits Tumor Growth and Reduces Interleukin-6 and Tumor Necrosis Factor α Levels in Rats with Walker 256 Carcinosarcoma." *Anticancer Research* 32, no. 1 (2012): 129–133. http://ar.iiarjournals.org/content/32/1/129.full.

Canani, Roberti Berni, Margherita Di Costanzo, Ludovica Leone, Monica Pedata, and Roasia Meli. "Potential Beneficial Effects of Butyrate in Intestinal and Extraintestinal Diseases." *World Journal of Gastroenterology* 17, no. 12 (2011): 1519–1528. www.ncbi.nlm.nih.gov /pmc/articles/PMC3070119/.

Center for Science in the Public Interest. "Why Good Nutrition Is So Important." Accessed October 1, 2019. https://cspinet.org/eating-healthy/why-good-nutrition-important.

Chainy, Gagan B. N., Sunil K. Manna, Madan M. Chaturvedi, and Bharat B. Aggarwai. "Anethole Blocks Both Early and Late Cellular Responses Transduced by Tumor Necrosis Factor: Effect on NF-κB, AP-1, JNK, MAPKK and Apoptosis." *Oncogene* 19 (2000): 2943–2950. www.nature.com/articles/1203614.

Chávez-Pesqueira, and Juan Núñez-Farfán Mariana. "Domestication and Genetics of Papaya: A Review." *Frontiers in Ecology and Evolution* 5 (2017): 1–9. doi:10.3389 /fevo.2017.00155.

Chattopadhyay, Ishita, Kaushik Biswas, Uday Bandyopadhyay, et al. "Turmeric and Curcumin: Biological Actions and Medicinal Applications." *Current Science* 87, no. 1 (2004): 44–53.

Chen, Shu-Qing, Ze-Shi Wang, Yi-Mao Ma, Wei Zhang, Jian-Liang Lu, Yue-Rong Liang, and Xin-Qiang Zheng. "Neuroprotective Effects and Mechanisms of Tea Bioactive Components in Neurodegenerative Diseases." *Molecules* 23, no. 3 (2018): 512–529. doi:10.3390 /molecules23030512.

Chevallier, Andrew. *Encyclopedia of Herbal Medicine: 550 Herbs and Remedies for Common Ailments*, 3rd ed. New York: DK Publishing, 2016.

Cleveland Clinic. "The Best Way You Can Get More Collagen." Accessed October 7, 2019. https://health.clevelandclinic.org/the-best-way-you-can-get-more-collagen/.

Cornell University. "Cooking Tomatoes Boosts Disease-Fighting Power." ScienceDaily. Accessed October 8, 2019. www.sciencedaily.com/releases/2002/04/020422073341.htm.

Crinnion, Walter J. "Organic Foods Contain Higher Levels of Certain Nutrients, Lower Levels of Pesticides, and May Provide Health Benefits for the Consumer." *Alternative Medicine Review* 15, no. 1 (2010): 4–12.

De Cassia da Silveria e Sa, Rita, Tamires Cardoso Lima, Flavio Rogerio de Nobrega, Anna Emmanuela Medeiros de Brito, and Damiao Pergentino de Sousa. "Analgesic-Like Activity of Essential Oil Constituents: An Update." *International Journal of Molecular Sciences* 18 (2017): 2392. www.ncbi.nlm.nih.gov/pmc/articles/PMC5751100/pdf/ijms-18-02392.pdf.

Diepvens, Kristel, Klass Westerterp, and Margriet Westerterp-Plantenga. "Obesity and Thermogenesis Related to the Consumption of Caffeine, Ephedrine, Capsaicin, and Green Tea." *American Journal of Physiology Regulatory, Integrative, and Comparative Physiology* 292, no. 1 (2007): R77–85. doi:10.1152/ajpregu.00832.2005.

Dincer, Cuneyt, Mert Karaoglan, Fidan Erden, et al. "Effect of Baking and Boiling on Nutritional and Antioxidant Properties of Sweet Potato (*Ipomoea batatas* [L.] Lam.) Cultivars." *Plant Foods for Human Nutrition* 66, no. 4 (2011): 341–347. https://link.springer.com/article/10.1007%2Fs11130-011-0262-0.

Farzaei, Mohammad Hosein, Zahra Abbasabadi, Mohammad Reza Shams Ardekani, Roja Rahimi, and Fatemeh Farzaei. "Parsley: A Review of Ethnopharmacology, Phytochemistry, and Biological Activities." *Journal of Traditional Chinese Medicine* 33, no. 6 (2013): 815–826. doi:10.1016/S0254-6272(14)60018-2.

Food and Agriculture Organization of the United Nations. "Traditional Crops: Moringa." Accessed October 3, 2019. www.fao.org/traditional-crops/moringa/en/.

Fuentes, Francisco, Ximena Paredes-Gonzalez, and Ah-Ng Tony Kong. "Dietary Glucosinolates Sulforaphane, Phenethyl Isothiocyanate, Indole-3-Carbinol/3,3'-Diindolylmethane: Anti-Oxidative Stress/Inflammation, Nrf2, Epigenetics/Epigenomics and *In Vivi* Cancer Chemopreventive Efficacy." *Current Pharmacology Reports* 1, no. 3 (2015): 179–196. doi:10.1007/s40495-015-0017-y.

Gil, Maria, Francisco Tomas-Barberan, Betty Hess-Pierce, Deirdre Holcroft, and Adel Kader. "Antioxidant Activity of Pomegranate Juice and Its Relationship with Phenolic Composition and Processing." *Journal of Agricultural and Food Chemistry* 48, no. 10 (2000): 4581–4589. doi:10.1021/jf000404a.

Gonzales, Gustavo. "Ethnobiology and Ethnopharmacology of *Lepidium meyenii* (Maca), a Plant from the Peruvian Highlands." *Evidence-Based Complementary and Alternative Medicine* (2012): 1–10. doi:10.1155/2012/193496.

Gullon, Beatriz, Patricia Gullon, Freni Tavaria, and Remedios Yanez. "Assessment of the Prebiotic Effect of Quinoa and Amaranth in the Human Intestinal Ecosystem." *Food & Function* 9, no. 7 (2016): 3782–3788. https://pubs.rsc.org/en/content/articlelanding /2016/FO/C6FO00924G#!divAbstract.

Hasanudin, Khairunnisa, Puziah Hashim, and Shuhaimi Mustafa. "Corn Silk (*Stigma Maydis*) in Healthcare: A Phytochemical and Pharmacological Review." *Molecules* 17, no. 8 (2012): 9697–9715. doi:10.3390/molecules17089697.

Heck, C. I., and E. G. De Mejia. "Yerba Mate Tea (*Ilex paraguariensis*): A Comprehensive Review on Chemistry, Health Implications, and Technological Considerations." *Journal of Food Science* 72, no. 9 (2007). doi:10.1111/j.1750-3841.2007.00535.x.

Hewlings, Susan, and Douglas Kalman. "Curcumin: A Review of Its Effects on Human Health." *Foods* 6, no. 10 (2017): 92. doi:10.3390/foods6100092.

Honda, Masaki, Hakuto Kageyama, Takashi Hibino, Ryota Takemura, Mononobu Goto, and Tetsuya Fukaya. "Enhanced Z-Isomerization of Tomato Lycopene Through the Optimal Combination of Food Ingredients." *Scientific Reports* 9 (2019): 1–7. doi:10.1038 /s41598-019-44177-4.

Huntley, Alyson L., Joanne Thompson Coon, and Edzard Ernst. "The Safety of Herbal Medicinal Products Derived from Echinacea Species." *Drug Safety* 28, no. 5 (2005): 387–400. doi:10.2165/00002018-200528050-00003.

Hvas, A.M., S. Juul, P. Bech, and E. Nexo. "Vitamin B_6 Level Is Associated with Symptoms of Depression." *Psychotherapy and Psychosomatics* 73 (2004): 340–343. doi:10.1159/000080386.

Irani, Morvarid, Malihe Amirian, Ramin Sadeghi, Junine Le Lez, and Robab Latifnejad Roudsari. "The Effect of Folate and Folate Plus Zinc Supplementation on Endocrine Parameters and Sperm Characteristics in Sub-Fertile Men: A Systematic Review and Meta-Analysis." *Urology Journal* 14, no. 5 (2017): 4069–4078. www.ncbi.nlm.nih.gov/pubmed/28853101.

Johri, R. K. "*Cuminum cyminum* and *Carum carvi*: An Update." *Pharmacognosy Review* 5, no. 9 (2011): 63–72. doi:10.4103/0973-7847.79101.

Joubert, E., and D. de Beer. "Rooibos (*Aspalathus linearis*) Beyond the Farm Gate: From Herbal Tea to Potential Phytopharmaceutical." *South African Journal of Botany* 77, no. 4 (2011): 869–886. doi:10.1016/j.sajb.2011.07.004.

Kahlon, T. S., M. H. Chapman, and G. E. Smith. "In Vitro Binding of Bile Acids by Spinach, Kale, Brussels Sprouts, Broccoli, Mustard Greens, Green Bell Pepper, Cabbage, and Collards." *Food Chemistry* 100, no. 4 (2007): 1531–1536. doi:10.1016/j.foodchem .2005.12.020.

Kato, Yoji, Tokio Domoto, Masanori Hiramitsu, et al. "Effects of Blood Pressure of Daily Lemon Ingestion and Walking." *Journal of Nutrition and Metabolism* (2014): 1–6. doi:10.1155/2014/912684.

Kaushik, Ujjwal, Vidhu Aeri, and Showkat R. Mir. "Cucurbitacins—An Insight into Medicinal Leads from Nature." *Pharmacognosy Review* 9, no. 17 (2015): 12–18. doi:10.4103/0973-7847.156314.

Kennedy, Pagan. "Who Made That Kale?" *New York Times*. Accessed October 8, 2019. www.nytimes.com/2013/10/20/magazine/who-made-that-kale.html.

Koulivand, Peir Hossein, Maryam Khaleghi Ghadiri, and Ali Gorji. "Lavender and the Nervous System." *Evidence-Based Complementary and Alternative Medicine.* (2013): 1–10. doi:10.1155/2013/681304.

Ku, Sae-Kwang, Soyoung Kwak, Yaesol Kim, and Jong-Sup Bae. "Aspalathin and Nothofagin from Rooibos (*Aspalathus linearis*) Inhibits High Glucose-Induced Inflammation *In Vitro* and *In Vivo*." *Inflammation* 38, no. 1 (2015): 445–455. doi:10.1007/s10753-014-0049-1.

Kujawska, Monika. "Yerba Mate (*Ilex paraguariensis*) Beverage: Nutraceutical Ingredient or Conveyor for the Intake of Medicinal Plants? Evidence from Paraguayan Folk Medicine." *Evidence-Based Complementary and Alternative Medicine* (2018). doi:10.1155/2018 /6849317.

Lachman, J., D. Miholova, V. Pivec, K. Jiru, and D. Janovska. "Content of Phenolic Anti-oxidants and Selenium in Grain of Einkorn (*Triticum monococcum*), Emmer (*Triticum dicoccum*), and Spring Wheat (*Triticum aestivum*) Varieties." *Plant, Soil, and Environment* 57, no. 5 (2011): 235–243. www.agriculturejournals.cz/publicFiles/40030.pdf.

Lippi, Donatella. "Chocolate in History: Food, Medicine, Medi-Food." *Nutrients* 5 (2013): 1573–1584. doi:10.3390/nu5051573.

Loren, David, Navindra Seeram, Risa Schulman, and David Holtzman. "Maternal Dietary Supplementation with Pomegranate Juice Is Neuroprotective in an Animal Model of Neonatal Hypoxic-Ischemic Brain Injury." *Pediatric Research* 57 (2005): 858–864. www.nature.com/articles/pr2005159.

Ludy, Mary-Jon, and Richard D. Mattes. "The Effects of Hedonically Acceptable Red Pepper Doses on Thermogenesis and Appetite." *Physiology & Behavior* 102, nos. 3–4 (2011): 251–258. doi:10.1016/j.physbeh.2010.11.018.

Lusby, P. E., A. Coombes, and J. M. Wilkinson. "Honey: A Potent Agent for Wound Healing?" *Journal of Wound, Ostomy, and Continence Nursing* 29, no. 6 (2002): 295–300. https://journals.lww.com/jwocnonline/Abstract/2002/11000/ Honey__A_Potent_Agent_for_Wound_Healing_.8.aspx?trendmd-shared=0.

Mahomoodally, M. Fawazi. "Traditional Medicines in Africa: An Appraisal of Ten Potent African Medicinal Plants." *Evidence-Based Complementary and Alternative Medicine* 2013. doi:10.1155/2013/617459.

Maia, L., A. De Mendonca. "Does Caffeine Intake Protect from Alzheimer's Disease?" *European Journal of Neurology* 9, no. 4 (2002). doi:10.1046/j.1468-1331.2002.00421.x.

Marnewick, Jeanine L., Fanie Rautenback, Irma Venter, Henry Neethling, Dee M. Blackhurst, Petro Wolmarans, and Muiruri Macharia. "Effects of Rooibos (*Aspalathus linearis*) on Oxidative Stress and Biochemical Parameters in Adults at Risk for Cardiovascular Disease." *Journal of Ethnopharmacology* 133, no. 1 (2011): 46–52. doi:10.1016/j .jep.2010.08.061.

Maxwell, Ellen G., Nigel J. Belshaw, Keith W. Waldron, and Victor J. Morris. "Pectin–An Emerging New Bioactive Food Polysaccharide." *Trends in Food Science & Technology* 24, no. 2 (2012): 64–73. https://doi.org/10.1016/j.tifs.2011.11.002.

McKay, Diane L., and Jeffrey B. Blumberg. "A Review of the Bioactivity and Potential Health Benefits of Peppermint Tea (*Mentha piperita* L.)." *Phytotherapy Research* 20, no. 8 (2006). doi:10.1002/ptr.1936.

Melese, Bethlehem, Neela Satheesh, Solomon WorknehFanta. "Emmer Wheat—An Ethiopian Prospective: A Short Review." *Annals. Food Science and Technology* 20, no. 1 (2019): 89–96. www.afst.valahia.ro/images/documente/2019/issue1/III.1_Melese.pdf.

Memorial Sloane Kettering Cancer Center. "D-limonene." Accessed October 9, 2019. www.mskcc.org/cancer-care/integrative-medicine/herbs/d-limonene.

Meng, Xiao, Ya Li, Sha Li, Yue Zhou, Ren-You Gan, Dong-Ping Xu, and Hua-Bin Li. "Dietary Sources and Bioactivities of Melatonin." *Nutrients* 9, no. 4 (2017): 367. doi:10.3390/nu9040367.

Momose, Yuko, Mari Maeda-Yamamoto, and Hiroshi Nabetani. "Systematic Review of Green Tea Epigalocatechin Gallate in Reducing Low-Density Lipoprotein Cholesterol Levels of Humans." *International Journal of Food Sciences and Nutrition* 67, no. 6 (2016): 606–613. doi:10.1080/09637486.2016.1196655.

Mursase, Takatoshi, Koichi Misawa, Satoshia Haramizu, Yoshihiko Minegishi, and Tadashi Hase. "Nootkatone, a Characteristic Constituent of Grapefruit, Stimulates Energy Metabolism and Prevents Diet-Induced Obesity by Activating AMPK." *American Journal of Physiology, Endocrinology, and Metabolism* 299, no. 2 (2010): E266–E275. doi:10.1152/ajpendo.00774.2009.

Murrary, Michael, and Joseph Pizzorno. *The Encyclopedia of Natural Medicine*. 3rd ed. New York: Atria, 2012.

Muruganantham, N., S. Solomon, and M. M. Senthamilselvi. "Anti-Cancer Activity of *Cucumis sativus* (Cucumber) Flowers Against Human Liver Cancer." *International Journal of Pharmaceutical and Clinical Research* 8, no. 1 (2016): 39–41. http://impactfactor.org/PDF/IJPCR/8/IJPCR,Vol8,Issue1,Article8.pdf.

Nathan, Pradeep J., Kristy Lu, Marcus Gray, and Christopher Oliver. "The Neuropharmacology of L-Theanine (N-Ethyl-L-Glutamine): A Possible Neuroprotective and Cognitive Enhancing Agent." *Journal of Herbal Pharmacotherapy* 6, no. 2 (2006): 21–30. www.ncbi.nlm.nih.gov/pubmed/17182482.

National Center for Complementary and Integrative Health. "Bromelain." September 2016. Accessed October 9, 2019. https://nccih.nih.gov/health/bromelain.

National Coffee Association. "NCA National Coffee Data Trends 2019." National Coffee Association. Accessed October 29, 2019. https://nationalcoffee.blog/2019/03/09/national-coffee-drinking-trends-2019/.

National Institutes of Health Office of Dietary Supplements. "Vitamin B_6 Fact Sheet for Health Professionals." Accessed October 3, 2019. https://ods.od.nih.gov/factsheets /VitaminB6-HealthProfessional/.

National Institutes of Health Office of Dietary Supplements. "Vitamin D Fact Sheet for Health Professionals." Accessed October 9, 2019. https://ods.od.nih.gov/factsheets /VitaminD-HealthProfessional/.

New World Encyclopedia. "Squash (Plant)." Accessed October 7, 2019. https://www .newworldencyclopedia.org/entry/squash_(plant).

Niaz, Kamal, Faheem Maqbool, Jaji Bahadar, and Mohammad Abdollahi. "Health Benefits of Manuka Honey as an Essential Constituent for Tissue Regeneration." *Current Drug Metabolism* 18, no. 10 (2017): 881–892. doi:10.2174/1389200218666170911152240.

Northern Australia Aboriginal Kakadu Plum Alliance. "Benefits of Kakadu Plum." Accessed September 30, 2019. https://naakpa.com.au/research.

The Nutrition Source. "Bananas." Harvard T. H. Chan School of Public Health. Accessed October 8, 2019. www.hsph.harvard.edu/nutritionsource/food-features/bananas/.

Ojansivu, Ilkka, Celia Lucia Ferreira, and Seppo Salminen. "Yacon, a New Source of Prebiotic Oligosaccharides with a History of Safe Use." *Trends in Food Science & Technology* 22, no. 1 (2011): 40–46. doi:10.1016/j.tifs.2010.11.005.

Oldways Whole Grains Council. "Quinoa—March Grain of the Month." *Wholegrainscouncil. org*. Accessed October 10, 2019. https://wholegrainscouncil.org/whole-grains-101 /grain-month-calendar/quinoa---march-grain-month.

Ooshima, T., T. Minami, W. Aono, Y. Tamura, and S. Hamada. "Reduction of Dental Plaque Deposition in Humans by Oolong Tea Extract." *Caries Research* 28 (1994): 146–149. doi:10.1159/000261636.

Patil B. S., and L. M. Pike. "Distribution of Quercetin Content in Different Rings of Various Coloured Onion (*Allium cepa* L.) Cultivars." *Journal of Horticultural Science* 70, no. 4 (1995): 643–650. doi:10.1080/14620316.1995.11515338.

Peana, A. T., P. S. D'Aquila, F. Panin, G. Serra, P. Pippia, and M.D. L. Moretti. "Anti-Inflammatory Activity of Linalool and Linalyl Acetate Constituents of Essential Oils." *Phytomedicine* 9, no. 8 (2002): 721–726. doi:10.1078/0944711023216213222.

Peterson, David, Martha Hahn, and Cheryl Emmons. "Oat Avenanthramides Exhibit Antioxidant Activities In Vitro." *Food Chemistry* 79, no. 4 (2002): 473–478. doi:10.1016 /S0308-8146(02)00219-4.

Pitchford, Paul. *Healing with Whole Foods: Asian Traditions and Modern Nutrition*. 3rd edition. Berkeley. CA: North Atlantic Books, 2002.

Popolo, Ada, Aldo Pinto, Maria Daglia, Seyed Fazel Nabavi, Ammad Ahmad Faroogi, and Luca Rastreeli. "Two Likely Targets for the Anticancer Effect of Indole Derivatives from Cruciferous Vegetables: PI3K/Akt/mTOR Signaling Pathway and the Aryl Hydrocarbon Receptor." *Seminars in Cancer Biology* 46 (2017): 132–137. doi:10.1016 /j.semcancer.2017.06.002.

Prasad, Sahdeo, and Bharat B. Aggarwal. *Turmeric, the Golden Spice: From Traditional Medicine to Modern Medicine*. In: Benzie IFF, S Wachtel-Galor, editors. *Herbal Medicine: Biomolecular and Clinical Aspects*. 2nd edition. Boca Raton: CRC Press/Taylor & Francis; 2011. Chapter 13. https://www.ncbi.nlm.nih.gov/books/NBK92752/.

Rao, Pasupuleti Visweawara, and Siew Hua Gan. "Cinnamon: A Multifaceted Medicinal Plant." *Evidence-Based Complementary and Alternative Medicine* 2014: 1–12. doi:10.1155/2014/642942.

Rilvin, Richard S. "Historical Perspective on the Use of Garlic." *The Journal of Nutrition* 131, no. 3 (2001): 951S–954S. doi:10.1093/jn/131.3.951S.

Sienkiewicz, Monika, Minika Lysakowska, Marta Pastuszka, Wojciech Bienias, and Edward Kowalczyk. "The Potential of Use Basil and Rosemary Essential Oils as Effective Antibacterial Agents." *Molecules* 18 (2013): 9334–9351. doi:10.3390/molecules18089334.

Srinivasan, Krishnapura. "Cumin *(Cuminum cyminum)* and Black Cumin (*Nigella sativa*) Seeds: Traditional Uses, Chemical Constituents, and Nutraceutical Effects." *Food Quality and Safety* 2, no. 1 (2018): 1–16. doi:10.1093/fqsafe/fyx031

Srinivasan, Krishnapura. "Ginger Rhizomes (*Zingiber officinale*): A Spice with Multiple Health Beneficial Potentials." *PharmaNutrition* 5, no. 1 (2017): 18–28. https:// www.researchgate.net/publication/312143507_Ginger_rhizomes_Zingiber_officinale _A_spice_with_multiple_health_beneficial_potentials.

Stahl, Wilhelm, and Helmut Sies. "β-Carotene and Other Carotenoids in Protection from Sunlight." *The American Journal of Clinical Nutrition* 96, no. 5 (2012) 1179S–1184S. doi:10.3945/ajcn.112.034819.

Street, Renée, Jasmeen Sidana, and Gerhard Prinsloo. "*Cichoium intybus*: Traditional Uses, Phytochemistry, Pharmacology, and Toxicology." *Evidence-Based Complementary and Alternative Medicine* (2013). doi:10.1155/2013/579319.

Tortorella, S. M., S. G. Royce, P. V. Licciardi, and T. C. Karagiannis. "Dietary Sulforaphane in Cancer Chemoprevention: The Role of Epigenetic Regulation and HDAC Inhibition." *Antioxidants & Redox Signaling* 22, no.16 (2015):1382–1424. doi:10.1089/ars.2014.6097.

Trinklein, David. "Cucumber: A Brief History." Integrated Pest Management University of Missouri. Accessed October 7, 2019. https://ipm.missouri.edu/MEG/2014/3/Cucumber-A-Brief-History/.

US Apple Association. "Popular Varieties." Accessed October 2, 2019. http://usapple.org/the-industry/apple-varieties/.

US Centers for Disease Control and Prevention. *Second National Report on Biochemical Indicators of Diet and Nutrition in the US Population 2012*. Accessed October 3, 2019. www.cdc.gov/nutritionreport/pdf/exesummary_web_032612.pdf.

US Department of Agriculture. "A Brief History of USDA Food Guides." Accessed October 3, 2019. www.choosemyplate.gov/eathealthy/brief-history-usda-food-guides.

US Department of Agriculture. FoodData Central "Avocados, Raw, All Commercial Varieties." Accessed October 9, 2019. https://fdc.nal.usda.gov/fdc-app.html#/food-details/171705/nutrients.

Vermeer, Cees. "Vitamin K: The Effect on Health Beyond Coagulation—An Overview." *Food & Nutrition Research* 56 (2012). www.ncbi.nlm.nih.gov/pmc/articles/PMC3321262/.

Wallace, Taylor, Robert Murray, and Kathleen Zelman. "The Nutritional Value and Health Benefits of Chickpeas and Hummus." *Nutrients* 8 (2016): 766. doi:10.3390/nu8120766.

Webb, Denise. "Anthocyanins." *Today's Dietitian 16, no. 3 (March 2014): 20*. Accessed October 7, 2019. https://www.todaysdietitian.com/newarchives/030314p20.shtml.

Weerawatanakorn, Monthana, Wei-Lun Hung, Min-Hsiung Pan, Shiming Li, Daxiang Li, Xiaochun Wan, and Chi-Tang Ho. "Chemistry and Health Beneficial Effects of Oolong Tea and Theasinensins." *Food Science and Human Wellness* 4, no. 4 (2015): 133–146. doi:10.1016/j.fshw.2015.10.002.

Williams, Cheryll. *Medicinal Plants in Australia Volume 3: Plants, Potions, and Poisons*. Australia: Rosenberg Publishing, 2012.

Yang, Yi-Ching, Feng-Hwa Lu, and Jin-Shang Wu. "The Protective Effect of Habitual Tea Consumption on Hypertension." *Archives of Internal Medicine* 164, no. 14 (2004): 1534–1540. www.ncbi.nlm.nih.gov/pubmed/15277285.

Yeager, Selene, and the Editors of *Prevention. The Doctors Book of Food Remedies*. New York: Rodale, 2007.

Zarfeshany, Aida, Sedigheh Asgary, and Shaghayegh Haghjoo Javanmard. "Potent Health Effects of Pomegranate." Advanced *Biomedical Research* 3, no.100 (2014). doi:10.4103/2277-9175.129371.

Zhang, Yan, Hang Ma, Weixi Liu, Tao Yuan, and Navindra P. Seeram. "New Antiglycative Compounds from Cumin (*Cuminum cyminum*) Spice." *Journal of Agricultural and Food Chemistry* 63 (2015): 10097–10102. doi:10.1021/acs.jafc.5b04796.

INDEX

HEALTH/MEDICAL CONDITION INDEX

M

Men's health
  chickpeas, 125–127
  pomegranates,
    95–98
Mood
  coffee, 172–173
  green tea, 174–175
  oolong, 176–177
Muscles and joints
  cayenne, 165–167
  farro, 114–118
  ginger, 159–161
  lavender, 150–152
  oranges, 71–73
  pumpkins, 59–61
  turmeric, 156–158

N

Nail health
  carrots, 24–26
  tomatoes, 62–64
Nausea
  acorn squash, 55–58
  bananas, 89–91
  cinnamon, 153–155
  ginger, 159–161
  lemons, 74–76
  mint, 138–140
Nerve function
  farro, 114–118
Neurodegenerative
  diseases
  coffee, 172–173
  oolong, 176–177

O

Obesity
  apples, 77–79
  broccoli, 52–54
  cauliflower, 49–51
  grapefruits, 68–70
  green tea, 174–175
  oolong, 176–177
Osteoporosis
  broccoli, 52–54
  brussels sprouts, 46–48
  pineapples, 80–82
  quinoa, 108–110

P

Pain
  cayenne, 165–167
  lavender, 150–152
  mint, 138–140
Pregnancy
  acorn squash, 55–58
  bananas, 89–91
  beets, 21–23
  broccoli, 52–54
  corn, 111–113
  ginger, 159–161
  grapefruits, 68–70
  lemons, 74–76
  lentils, 119–121
  parsley, 146–148
  parsnips, 27–30
  peas, 131–133
  pomegranates, 95–98
  spinach, 37–39
Psoriasis
  turmeric, 156–158

R

Respiratory infections
  mint, 138–140

S

Skin health
  almonds, 128–130
  avocados, 83–85
  blueberries, 86–88
  carrots, 24–26
  grapefruits, 68–70
  lavender, 150–152
  oats, 105–107
  pumpkins, 59–61
  tomatoes, 62–64
  watermelons, 92–94
Stamina
  beets, 21–23
Stress
  bananas, 89–91

T

Thyroid health
  brown rice, 102–104

W

Weight loss/management
  almonds, 128–130
  apples, 77–79
  avocados, 83–85
  beets, 21–23
  black beans, 122–124
  blueberries, 86–88
  brown rice, 102–104
  cauliflower, 49–51
  cayenne, 165–167

ACKNOWLEDGMENTS

Thank you to my incredible husband (and best friend): Your constant encouragement, love, and support mean the world. It really is "all good," babe! To my Harper bean: Your curiosity and happiness inspire me daily. Keep on giggling and never stop exploring!

Dad, thank you for being my steadfast cheerleader. Mom, you've taught me to aim high and never give up on my dreams. Thank you both for sharing your love of cooking with me. Farley, you're simply the best in so many ways. You embody what it means to be a good sister and an even better friend.

To my extended family (especially Jan who is Gaga-extraordinaire!) and friends, your encouragement and support of my nutrition pursuits are truly incredible.

To all the amazing dietitians I've worked alongside, especially Stephanie, Joy, Pegah, and Sydney, thank you for being sources of inspiration in the field.

Thank you to the Callisto Media team and my wonderful editor, Crystal Nero. You've helped make my dream of becoming an author come true.

ABOUT THE AUTHOR

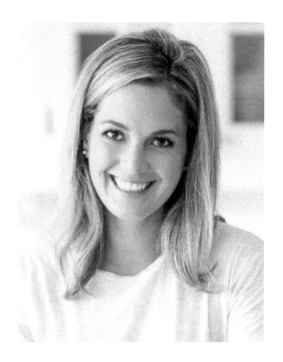

Eliza Savage, RD, MS, CDN, is a registered dietitian with a lifelong passion for wellness. She has extensive experience counseling patients one on one in private practice and in outpatient settings at New York City's top hospitals. As a nutritionist, she writes for various wellness companies, consults with brands as a nutrition expert, and contributes to media outlets such as Women's Health, Well+Good, and Health. With a background in marketing, Eliza combines her love of writing with her comprehensive nutrition knowledge to create approachable and straightforward content. When not working, Eliza is running in Central Park, strolling with her daughter, or testing recipes with her husband. Connect with Eliza at www.ElizaSavageNutrition.com or follow her on Instagram @ElizaSavageNutrition.